JIU–JITSU

and

SELF DEFENSE

Moshe Feldenkrais

Moti Nativ

Genesis II Publishing, Inc.

Longmont, Colorado

Jiu-Jitsu and Self Defense

Moshe Feldenkrais (1904-1984)

Moti Nativ

Jiu-Jitsu and Self Defense / by Moshe Feldenkrais © 1930

Published by:
Genesis II Publishing, Inc.
AchievingExcellence.com
Longmont, Colorado, USA

Designer: Al Wadleigh

LCCN: 2021944126

ISBN-13: 978-1-884605-21-5 (ebook)
ISBN-13: 978-1-884605-11-6

Printed in USA

"The reader who closely examines the tactics shown in this book will realize that the beginning of each technique is the instinctive movement a person makes when he is attacked in the manner described... Therefore, the defender doesn't have to determine how to begin before he actually begins; starting comes by itself, instinctively."

– Moshe Feldenkrais, Tel Aviv, 1930

CONTENTS

Part 2

PREFACE

TO THE NEW EDITION

by Moti Nativ

The first time I got up on stage to introduce the book *Jiu-Jitsu and Self Defense* to the public was in 2004, at an event commemorating Moshe Feldenkrais's centennial birthday. My martial arts students and I demonstrated techniques from the book that evening.

I love to search for rare books on martial arts in used book stores in Tel Aviv. I walked into a store that I frequented and the seller, who recognized me from previous visits, opened a well-hidden drawer. In that drawer, he pulled out *Jiu-Jitsu and Self Defense* by Moshe Feldenkrais. It turned out to be a first edition copy with a handwritten dedication to a friend of Moshe's. There was another treasure hiding between the pages—the original passport photo that was used for the front piece! The photo led to a photography studio where I garnered a few more details about Moshe's life. The book was expensive, but I didn't hesitate, and it has been my companion ever since.

In 2008, I purchased the rights to translate this book from Michel Feldenkrais Silice.

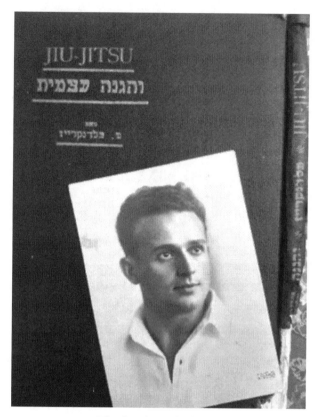

The book and photo.

I began work on this project quite energetically. However, circumstances (both professional and health-related) stalled this project and now, in 2020, I am ready to bring it to fruition. During the intervening years, I have had to deal with a few medical issues. The *Feldenkrais Method®* helped me to rehabilitate myself and overcome these health problems.

It is said that "every delay is for the good." My body and brain have been through a lot during the past years and I have clarified many insights, discoveries, and new connections. I feel that now is the optimal time to write this preface and, furthermore, I must restrain myself because I could write an entire book *about* this book.

I found that returning to work on the English version of this book in the year 2020 had special significance because this year we commemorate the Haganah's centenary. The Haganah was a Jewish paramilitary organization, which sixteen-year-old Moshe Feldenkrais joined at its inception in 1920. Ten years later, this book describing his training method, which was based on a decade of field experience, was published. More than a decade has passed since I began this project. During the intervening years, I developed a deep, personal connection to this book and to Moshe, the martial artist. This book spurred me to research the synergy between the *Feldenkrais Method* and martial arts. I have taught over three hundred workshops, which grew out of this synergy.

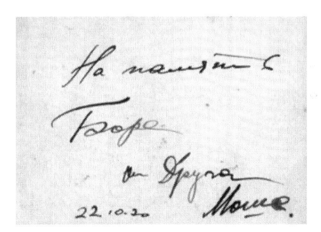

Dedication written in Russian.

We tend to consider Moshe a genius because of his *Awareness Through Movement*® (ATM®) lessons. However, I contend that his genius was evident much before he developed the method that bears his name. I claim that *Jiu-Jitsu and Self Defense* was its first blossom.

After many years of studying martial arts and engaging in intensive training sessions, which were often quite extreme, in hindsight, I stupidly pushed myself with no regard to my limits; I had a body that had sustained many injuries. My knees had suffered considerable injury. These injuries were due to the soccer that I played early on, like Moshe. A back injury during Judo training in 1985 brought me to the point where the orthopedists recommended that I stop training and undergo surgery to correct an extreme displacement of the L4-L5 vertebrae. As I was readying myself for surgery, I was introduced to the *Feldenkrais Method* by my sensei, Doron Navon. After a number of *Functional Integration®* lessons with Jeremy Krauss, I joined an ATM group led by Eli Wadler. I was the only man in the early morning class. I was strong and young and you can imagine my surprise when I saw that my fellow students, who were all elderly women, performed the movements easily and gracefully while I struggled. After the lesson, I was astonished to discover that I remembered the entire movement sequence. I wrote down all the steps of the lesson and began to teach these movement lessons to my martial arts students. For a long time, I went to an ATM lesson each morning and taught the same lesson during the evening martial arts training. Uli Yaron, a *Feldenkrais Method* practitioner, who happened to be present when I was teaching a movement lesson at my dojo, encouraged me to enroll in a *Feldenkrais* Professional Training Program (FPTP).

In 1991, I registered for the FPTP Jerusalem 1 (Anat Ban-
iel, Educational Director) and graduated in 1994. I had
had quite a bit of practical experience by the time I start-
ed the practitioner training course, but that didn't really
give me an advantage over the other trainees. Each one
brought his or her unique talents and we all went through
a learning process that yielded wonderful results. One
thing that I felt was lacking in my course (and apparently in other FPTPs also) was the historical background of
Feldenkrais, the martial artist himself. Truthfully, even
though I am a martial artist, I did not pay attention to
this lacuna at the time. When I completed my course, I
still had my day job and did not have the time to develop a full-time *Feldenkrais* practice. However, I continued
teaching ATM lessons during training sessions with my
martial arts students. Through my research, I came to
understand that Moshe's first students of the *Feldenkrais
Method* were *judokas* and British soldiers stationed at an
army base in Scotland, where he was contributing to the

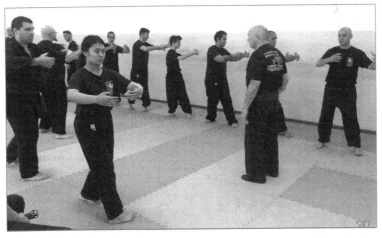

*Teaching the ATM Lesson, "Turning on the Heels" in Club
Kim Long, Milan.*

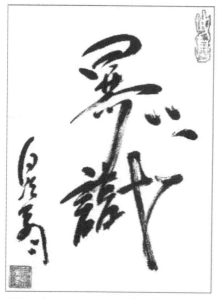

Warrior Awareness (Calligraphy: Masaaki Hatsumi)

British war effort as a scientist.

When I teach ATM lessons as part and parcel of martial arts training, it is not to simply teach lessons to improve self-awareness, but rather to use elements of the lessons as warm-ups in preparation for the training sessions. I teach specific movements or techniques needed to improve both physical action and survival skills.

I have exposed my students to ATM lessons at different stages of their development in the martial arts, so they have also acquired knowledge that they then passed on to their students. My Japanese teacher, Dr. Masaaki Hatsumi, realized that the issue of awareness was a central element in my approach. He awarded my dojo the name "shiki" (awareness) and thus my dojo is called "Warrior Awareness" (Mu-I-Shiki).

My research unearthed the significant fact that Feldenkrais developed the first Israeli self-defense method, which he published as *Jiu-Jitsu and Self Defense*. I was pleased and proud to have discovered this, but I was also angry that the Krav Maga community didn't appreciate Feldenkrais's contribution to the development of Israeli martial arts. To rectify this, I lecture about Feldenkrais in Krav Maga instructors' advanced trainings at Wingate Institute. I made sure that Feldenkrais's self-defense method is mentioned in *Kapap – From the Field to the Battlefield* (published by Noah Gross, 2010), which describes the development of Israeli hand-to-hand combat methods. I jumped at the opportunity to write the foreword to a Krav Maga instructors manual (Guy Mor and Abi Moriya, 2016) where I detailed other aspects of Feldenkrais's self-defense method. I collaborated with my friend and student Noah Gross in writing the chapter about the development of Krav Maga, which appears in a book about the history of the Israeli Defense Forces (IDF) Division of Combat Fitness (2018). I emphasized the fact that Feldenkrais was the first in Palestine-Eretz Yisrael[1] to develop a self-defense method and, maybe more importantly, effective training techniques. In his academic article *The Case for the Recognition of Krav Maga as Part of the Intangible Cultural Heritage of Israel* (Scientific Research, Vol.7 No.4, April 2019), Dr. Guy Mor quoted my foreword from *Thinking and Doing*[2], "Feldenkrais (1904-1984), who had experience in Jiu-Jitsu and other hand-to-hand combat systems, sought to create a practical and more effective solution based on his own research. In doing so, he was incorporating the principle of "unconscious reaction" (also known as "reflexive reaction"). This approach is predicated on the assumption that human beings have a pre-programmed system of reactions to menaces and that these reactions are performed unconsciously. This insight led Feldenkrais to establish an improved fighting and training regimen whose fundamental principles were later adopted by both Kapap (an acronym of Krav Panim el Panim, meaning "hand-to-hand combat")[3] and Krav Maga (the modern Israeli martial art)."

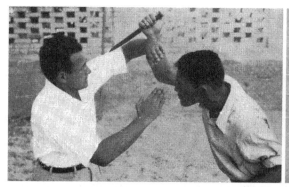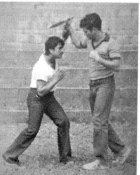

Defense against a knife attack Left: Moshe training with a partner, Right :Eli Avikzar Krav Maga (1968).[4]

As I got deeper into my research, I found it incumbent upon me to relate the history of Moshe, the martial artist, within the *Feldenkrais* community. I didn't want my research to come across as a story, but in a practical way through my teaching. After I retired from my job as head of Information Systems Division in the state comptroller's office in 2008, I began teaching workshops titled, *The Synergy of the Feldenkrais Method and the Martial Arts*. These workshops were geared to *Feldenkrais* practitioners, but martial artists were also welcome. Just as many other teachers bring what makes them unique to their *Feldenkrais* teaching, I also teach in a way that is distinctive to me.

Three unique things characterize my teaching. First, I am an active martial artist. Second, I have unique insights into rehabilitation through my personal experience. I have dealt with how to function with knee injuries, how to recover from back pain, how to regain confidence in one's body and its abilities, both mentally and physically. Thirdly, my expertise gained through extensive research into the roots of the *Feldenkrais Method* and how the martial arts influenced Moshe's thinking and doing.

It has also bothered me that the *Feldenkrais* community is, on the whole, not cognizant that Moshe's many years of martial arts training and teaching contained the seeds of what is known today as the *Feldenkrais Method*. I am confident that my argument, along with the evidence that I uncovered, will convince the reader that *Jiu-Jitsu and Self Defense* should be considered the first step toward the development of the *Feldenkrais Method*.

As for me, I never did have that back surgery. I just continued improving and discovering more about Moshe, the martial artist. I have mentioned a few parallels between my path in life and Moshe's. He grew up in the Land of Israel, as did I; he spoke Hebrew, as do I; we both suffered knee injuries during soccer games. He was a martial artist, as am I.

In 1950, at the age of forty-six, he returned to Israel and served as the head of the electronics department in the Israeli Defense Force's science division, leaving martial arts behind. However, he was still preoccupied with his Judo experience and his theories about mature behavior. No wonder that after three years in the IDF, Moshe retired to civilian life and dedicated himself to develop and promote *Awareness Through Movement*.

Thanks to the *Feldenkrais Method*, I am still teaching and studying martial arts at the age of seventy. I have been an active martial artist since 1966 and have taught martial arts for thirty-four years. My battered body continues to improve and here I am, a real-life example attesting to the efficacy of the *Feldenkrais Method*.

FOREWORD

TO THE NEW EDITION

by Moti Nativ

The Haganah was established one hundred years ago. The pioneer Moshe Feldenkrais joined the Haganah at the age of sixteen, actively helping defend the Jewish population from threats. Ten years of experience in hand-to-hand combat spurred Moshe to publish a book that presented an unusual self-defense method, which he designed. "I wrote a book which was intended for the Haganah based on all such movements of self-defense; where the first movement is the natural movement that you'll do without thinking, without knowing; anybody, any silly ass would do that to begin with."[5]

I contend that this handbook conceals something much more important than just demonstrating self-defense techniques. How many self-defense books contain a chapter entitled "How to Rescue Your Brother," which is dedicated to helping a friend in dire straits? Who else will suggest that you read a book by Sigmund Freud to gain a deeper understanding of fear? I maintain that this book contains the seeds that many decades later, grew into the *Feldenkrais Method*. I am even bold enough to suggest that Moshe's unique approach to self-defense training is the first *Feldenkrais Method*.

Feldenkrais opens with words reminding the reader that humility, mutual support in the learning process, commitment to spreading the knowledge, and safety (even toward enemies) are necessary for self-defense training, especially for making peace. The foreword begins with the quote, "If I am not for myself, who then is for me?"[6] Those words reveal Moshe's state of mind. Living in an environment where there was a constant threat of attack on Jewish enclaves lead him to develop his fighting method.

We cannot ignore the historical period of Moshe's youth in Tel Aviv, where the young pioneer struggled daily for his survival. Feldenkrais arrived in the Land of Israel in 1919 with the first group of the Third Aliya.[7] Living conditions were primitive. Many olim (immigrants on aliya to the Land of Israel) lived in tents pitched in the sands of the future city of Tel Aviv.

Needless to say, there was no electricity or refrigeration. Moshe fell ill from eating spoiled food and was hospitalized for an extended period.

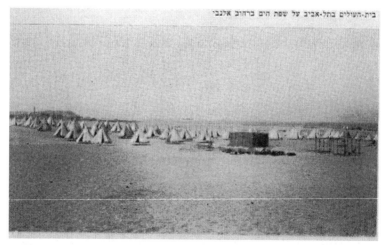

New immigrants living in tents where Tel Aviv stands today.

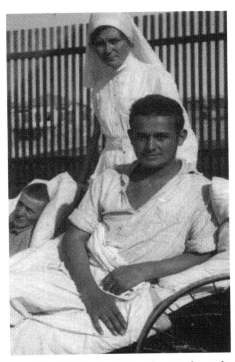

Moshe Feldenkrais in the Hadassah Hospital, Tel Aviv.

The most common and important work available at the time was in construction, building houses and roads. Feldenkrais joined the Baranovich construction group.

Hard labor strengthened his body, as we see from this description by Avigdor Grinspan in the book, *The Third Aliya.* "My teacher on the site was a former pupil of mine named Moshe Feldenkrais. He was a young boy, around 16 years old, broad-shouldered, and sturdy as an oak."

In May 1921, Arabs staged coordinated attacks on Jews in Tel Aviv and other communities. Forty-seven Jews were slaughtered and one hundred and forty-six were wounded. These attacks changed the relationship between Arabs and Jews, motivating the need for self-defense training.

This book describes a self-defense method for confronting the existential threats that were prevalent in the Land of Israel during this period. The book defines techniques and ideas for self-defense training. It was considered a fairly good book in those days, which could compete with the many martial arts books on the market. Today, knowing that Moshe developed his eponymous

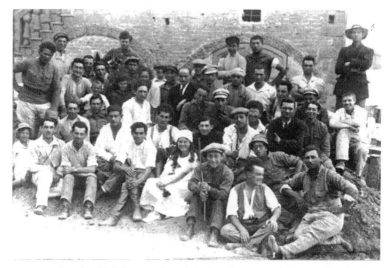

Moshe Feldenkrais with the Baranovich group.

method adds another layer when considering the book's contents. We may find some clues hinting at the foundational principles of the future *Feldenkrais Method*. Even more significant for us, this book allows us a glimpse of Moshe's talents and personality, showing the strength and dedication needed to create and promote the *Feldenkrais Method*.

Feldenkrais published two significant books over his decade in Tel Aviv, *Autosuggestion* and *Jiu-Jitsu and Self Defense*. These books are the work of a man growing from teenager to adult, one who struggled against sickness, poverty, and terror threats, while working, educating, and creating.

His words on the first edition of *Autosuggestion* (1929) tell us about his potent state of mind, "You've seen me in my poverty and this is the beginning of my might." Moshe was in top physical and mental condition. He had developed a self-defense method, leaving a manual for training

Haganah recruits. In that same time, he was making his final preparations to continue his studies in Paris.

The young Haganah recruit, Moshe Feldenkrais, engaged in hand-to-hand combat and saw many Haganah fighters injured and even killed during these clashes.

Feldenkrais was disappointed with the outcome of these confrontations. He was filled with sorrow at the loss of close friends killed in those fights. He could not bear the stinging defeats that the pioneers suffered in spite of having trained in Jiu-Jitsu. His disappointment was so deep that he even ventured to say that it would have been prefer-

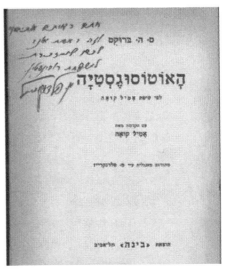

Cover page of Autosuggestion with Moshe Feldenkrais' signature.

able not to know Jiu-Jitsu because then his fellow fighters would be more likely to run away and escape with their lives. Moshe understood that the Jiu-Jitsu training did not prepare them for real combat situations. In the famous autobiographical interview in Amherst, June 1981, Moshe recounted, "I found out that the old form of Jiu-Jitsu didn't work. So, I set out to make Jiu-Jitsu of my own that will work."

Questioning the efficacy of the training, Moshe applied himself to developing his own method. Moshe surmised that if a person has to think too much about the movement, they are dead before they can move. He came up with an idea "...I built a system of defense for any sort of attack where the first movement is not what you think of doing, what you decide to do, but what you actually do when you are frightened. I said, all right, let's see now, we will train the people so that end of their first spontaneous movement is where we must start."[8]

He concluded that a self-defense system must be based on the instinctive movements a person makes when attacked. Even if a person does not train regularly, the spontaneous action awakens the body to complete the defensive movement. "Experience shows that the moment a person feels the touch of the aggressor's body on one of his limbs, he is freed from his momentary paralysis and he performs the whole trick with the same ease as in training, perhaps even better." This was the core concept of his self-defense method and the catalyst for writing this book.

Moshe referred to this phenomenon in the appendices to his Hebrew translation of *Autosuggestion* by Emil Coué: "The most effective protective movement pattern became determined and fixed so that it takes place despite of our conscious will."

He explained the advantage of this approach, "The reader who closely examines the tactics shown in this book will realize that the beginning of each technique is the instinctive movement a person makes when he is attacked in the manner described... Therefore, the defender doesn't have to determine how to begin before he actually begins; starting comes by itself, instinctively."

This concept assures that even after a long break in training the skill, will not be lost and learning will also be faster. "Practice shows that a comparatively short period of training is amply sufficient to learn how to continue the counter, which was already begun, and how to carry it out effectively."[9]

> *"...I built a system of defense for any sort of attack where the first movement is not what you think of doing, what you decide to do, but what you actually do when you are frightened."*
>
> – Moshe Feldenkrais, D.Sc., 1977

In the Introduction to Part 1, Feldenkrais predicts what thoughts and questions may occur to his readers. I liked Moshe's "answer" to the question about the danger of revealing the techniques to criminals: "I will reveal a secret known by all; the exercises and techniques in this book were actually thought up by the criminals themselves."[10]

We should credit Moshe for his commitment to safety during training. He mentions it in the introduction and flags the more dangerous techniques throughout the book: "The reader will find many techniques here that are marked as dangerous. Caution must be used. The reader must keep this in mind and only use these [dangerous] ploys when there is no other choice... Too strong a pull or using force beyond measure can harm the person training with you and cause him terrible injury."

Surprisingly, a self-defense method meant for training Haganah fighters starts with "Tricks to Use Against Rapists." I assume that Moshe was concerned about threats to Jewish women in Tel Aviv of those days and had no gender bias when it came to teaching how to fight.

His approach to using common objects as weapons is most important for anyone living in a dangerous environment. "Every object or non-object can serve as an excellent weapon against an attacker." You'll find a variety of examples of objects in the chapter devoted to weaponizing whatever is handy. Non-object is another pearl of Moshe's wisdom. I invite you to use your imagination and describe the non-objects that may rescue someone under attack. This idea was also dictated by time and place; the British Mandatory government forbade Jews from carrying firearms.

I find it important to mention that Moshe did not actually have a sensei[11] at that time. My own experience in Bujinkan Dojo, and that of my colleagues in different martial arts, is through many years of systematic learning under a sensei. Moshe described his Jiu-Jitsu instructor. "He studied Jiu-Jitsu in Berlin with one of the instructors of the police ...he was a man about twenty or twenty-one, a young boy, he taught that thing to us, as the members of the Haganah... and I worked with him."[12] This shows that Moshe's theory of self-defense was not rooted in the "normal" process of learning from an experienced teacher. It was a creation of Moshe's young mind and body responding to the situation of his community; based on his own experience and imagination. He wrote this book in a particular historical context, however, the universal application of the principles expounded here, makes it a timeless text.

Shortly after *Jiu-Jitsu and Self Defense* was published, Feldenkrais left Palestine-Eretz Yisrael to continue his education in France. According to him, one of the reasons he chose to leave at that particular time was that he feared how the British authorities would react to his book. Feldenkrais did not return to his homeland until after WWII. However, this book informed the development of KAPAP[13], an Israeli martial art. The following photo shows how Moshe's basic technique against a knife stab, a move performed by Moshe Hurvitz, the team leader who developed KAPAP. After the Israeli state was established, the IDF adopted the KAPAP method, which was renamed Krav Maga a few years later.

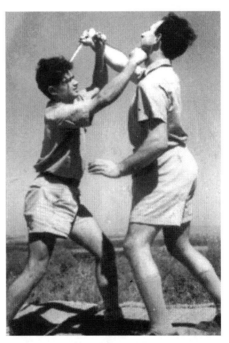

Apparently, after meeting Jigoro Kano in France, Moshe wrote a French version of this book which was published in 1934. For the French edition, Moshe changed the name of the book to *Jiu-Jitsu, La Defense du Faible Contre L'Agressur*.[14] Professor Kano wrote an introduction to this book, stating that it was the best book written on the subject outside of Japan.

Moshe Hurvitz demonstrating a basic defense against a knife attack, based on Moshe Feldenkrais' approach.

Moshe translated the original book into English, adding new material and restructuring the chapters. However, this edition was never published. In the preface of the draft version, he explains the background for the original book: "This book was originally conceived in an oriental[15] country where public security is not a very permanent institution and has periodical low tides. Whence the essentially practical character of these pages."

In the introduction to his book *Judo: The Art of Defense and Attack*,[16] he recounts that he had approached an English publisher and proposed publishing an English version of his original *Jiu-Jitsu* book. Being well-acquainted with Moshe's cunning, it has occurred to me that he already had an English version in hand. The publisher was not interested, but he commissioned Moshe to write a new book on Judo. My assumption proved correct when I tracked down an English version in the Kodokan[17] in Tokyo. My first thought was that Moshe had written this version just before he met the English publisher. However, after meticulously scrutinizing the document and reviewing what is known about his connection with Jigoro Kano, I concluded that the English draft

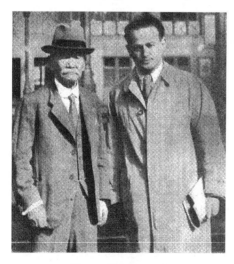

was written while Moshe was still in Paris; about two years after the French version was published. In September 1936, Kano returned to Paris for the occasion of opening the Jiu-Jitsu Club de France, co-founded by Moshe Feldenkrais.

Jigoro Kano and Moshe Feldenkrais, Paris 1936.

On this occasion Moshe handed his English draft to Kano. However, soon after, Kano passed away.

This document made its way to the Kodokan, but it is still not known whether Moshe received any feedback from Kano.

In 1941, after the English publisher rejected his proposal, Moshe abandoned his plan to publish an English edition of *Jiu-Jitsu*. The original English manuscript is now part of the Kodokan archives. Visitors to the archives can view a photocopy of the original. However, when I visited the Kodokan in 2009, the curator allowed me to see the original. It is interesting to note that Moshe suggested a change of title for the English edition. Two interesting options appear on the original binding: *Science Versus Brute Force* or *Jiu-Jitsu for Intellectuals*.

The book that you are now holding in your hands is a translation of the Hebrew version that was dedicated to the Jewish pioneers defending the Land of Israel. When comparing the French version, the never-published English manuscript, and the original Hebrew, it is apparent that Moshe did not make many changes in the contents of the book beyond reordering the chapters. The slight changes that were made reflect his development as a martial artist, his exposure to Judo, the philosophical mind-body approach, and the insights he gained living in a new environment, is shown in these pages.

Moshe demonstrates a wide range of techniques and explains concepts of self-defense by describing dangerous situations. He talks about the content and sources. "The reader will find in this book the best tricks of Jiu-Jitsu, permitting any man of average strength to defend himself against an armed aggressor of greater strength than himself. He will equally find a certain number of blows used by boxers, especially those which are most efficient and easiest to learn." Proudly, but with a hint of humility, Moshe writes, "...and finally some techniques which are the fruit of the author's experience as a teacher and of his imagination. Many of the tactics in this book originate in the wrestling style known as Catch-as-Catch-Can[18] and also those which I developed myself through teaching and research." In addition to writing about and demonstrating techniques, Moshe focuses on the importance of the mental elements and the psychology of self-defense.

Some salient points are:

Changing attitude

> "The critical moment is the one when a man, all unawares, is suddenly called to defend himself or attack somebody. If he is not seized with fright at that moment, the passage from the normal attitude to one of defense is instantaneous and without complication. But that is not what generally happens."

Freeing oneself from being petrified and paralyzed by fright

> Moshe explains the importance of "moving," "laughing," "breathing," and "posing." He emphasizes "moving" as the most important reaction. "The movements of the body have, indeed, exactly the same influence as the movements of the soul. Hence it is only necessary to break the ice with some movement in order to dissipate the torpor in which you may find yourself when attacked."

> Relating to laughing, Moshe quotes Professor James,[19] "We do not cry because we are sad, but we are sad because we cry." He continues with Goethe's

advice to laugh without any reason for doing so because laughter in itself brings forth gaiety.

Regarding "breathing" and "posing" Moshe advised: "It is best to combine a deep inhalation with some useful movement, such as putting yourself in the classical boxing posture, or simply clenching your fists and standing on your tiptoes, the rest of the body being entirely relaxed. Assume this "pose," even if your heart is not in it, you will be astonished to see how quickly your mood changes. In brief, try it, however ridiculous it may seem to you, and you will find that it works." Moshe suggests exploring the *Autosuggestion* method: "Those who are particularly interested in the question may read with great profit: *L'autosuggestion* by Charles Baudoin, *Le Maîtrise de Soi-même* by Émile Coué, and *The Nervous Temperament* by Adler."

Loyalty to friends and taking responsibility

This book was born into the reality of pioneers defending their homes, friends, ideology, and their very lives. It is impossible to ignore its historical context and Moshe's way of thinking. In doing so, he chose to include a chapter called "How to Rescue Your Brother," which reveals his unique *weltanschauung* (a German word that means world view), where the first goal should be to help a friend.

Conflict resolution

The second chapter in this book is about making peace (stopping fights). It may have been naïve, but Moshe intended to show how to prevent or de-escalate a quarrel between adversaries.

Principles of learning

> Along with the self-defense techniques and practical
> advice for survival, learning was already germane to
> Moshe's approach. We see him emphasizing two-sided
> exercising, training relaxation and exertion, learning
> conditions and the learning environment, haste is not
> speed, and other subjects related to the learning pro-
> cess. As we explore his writings on these topics, we
> will find that the ideas sowed here came to full flower
> in his later writings about the *Feldenkrais Method*.

Falls and falling was an important topic for Moshe. He
dedicates an entire chapter to the subject. He begins the
chapter titled *Falling*, by stating simply and clearly, "First
of all, one ought to learn how to fall correctly, without
hurting oneself."

Moshe stresses, "Special care should be taken to master
the forward and backward falls... They occur in everyday
life, as well. I myself was saved from death twice, thanks to
knowing how to fall." Moshe's personal remark reinforces
the fact that he wrote this book from practical experience.

To clarify matters, I think that I should point out that although Moshe uses the term "falling," he teaches backward and forward rolling in this chapter.

Here we get a glimpse of the author's personal integri-
ty. He writes, "The plates in this chapter show a correct
method of falling." To the discerning eye, there is a direct
evolutionary line from the chapter on falling to the ATM
lesson, *Head under a Frame* (Alexander Yanai Lessons #132
and #133), which teaches rolling in a wonderful way, giving the novice a process for learning how to roll and of-

fering the experienced judoka a way to improve his or her falling technique.

Feldenkrais clearly states the advantages of knowing how to fall:[20]

- Preserve oneself from injury
- Move away from the aggressor
- Free oneself from certain holds
- Use the power (momentum) of the fall to come back to standing
- Use the fall to cause the adversary an even worse fall

In a short chapter titled, "Blows (punches) and their Defense," Moshe brilliantly presented the essence of boxing. The variety of sources quoted show that he was quite knowledgeable about boxing. Emil Avineri,[21] a regional boxing champion and Feldenkrais' sparring partner, cooperated with Moshe on this book and appears in most of the photos. Feldenkrais was an avid fan of boxing and wrote, "When the agile, quick, and confident person (who may be weak in physical strength, but not in spirit), challenges and attacks the bulky giant, we can surmise that the victory will go to the attacker." His love of boxing is echoed in the San Francisco training where he talks about the fight between Baer and Carnera:[22] "You heard of Carnera, the boxer, here in America? Well, he was something, and then came Baer who was half his weight, and made a mess of him. It's not a question of size; it's a question of the quality of action. You can be very strong and worth nothing, and you can be agile and know what you're doing and you can do anything."[23]

He explains the body organization for an effective punch in his unique way:

"A straight left punch ought to be thrown so that all the joints interposed between the knuckles of the left fist and the right toe form no angle, so far as possible, the connecting bones being the straight extension of one another."

"To make this punch effective, the fist should be thrown as if it were a massive body, the arm being an articulated bar, or somewhat like a stone at the end of a string, i.e., the shoulder articulation is very free and without tightening the biceps."

"A good punch ought to smash the spot without pushing the whole body. And this quality of the punch is due principally to the velocity. When a good boxer works on the punching bag, every punch leaves an impression of the fist, making the bag swing only imperceptibly, all the power of the punch being absorbed by the local deformation. However, a novice working at the bag pushes it and sets it swaying like a pendulum."

"The right-handed punch is generally employed as a means of deciding the fight and is produced without other movements of the body, except those which directly engender the punch, so that there is nothing to impair the precision. The right-handed punch also ought to begin in the right toe."

We can find quite a few ATMs that Moshe developed this method to teach this body organization. Some relevant ATM lessons that deal with the connections and synchronization of legs and arms are Alexander Yanai #300 *In Standing, Turning the Heels Outside*, Alexander Yanai #373 *Turning on the Heels*, San Francisco training *On the Side, Reaching the Ceiling*.

I believe that this book would not have been written with–

out Moshe's practical fighting experience and the reality in which he lived. Moshe Feldenkrais was a physically strong man and a determined fighter, but he wrote this guide for the ordinary person who, by paying attention to the practical advice, can achieve effective performance of the techniques.

The original Hebrew version has ramifications for the development of what is known today as the *Feldenkrais Method*. According to Moshe's biography, this book was the catalyst for his meeting Kano and his involvement in the world of Judo, which was ultimately a source of inspiration and the testing ground for the development and structure of the *Feldenkrais Method*.

I am pleased with the opportunity to bring to fruition Moshe's wish of publishing an English edition of this vital document.

I chose to include this photo of Moshe in a "superman" stance, reaching to the sky. For me, it exemplifies this period of his life.

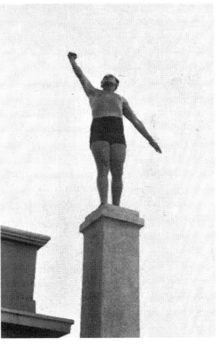

Moshe Feldenkrais, Tel Aviv, circa 1930.

Note from the Translator

More than a decade ago, Moti Nativ approached me about translating a fairly obscure book, which Moshe Feldenkrais published in 1930. He warned me that I might find the language a bit difficult because the Hebrew written by Moshe in the 1920s is quite different than the Hebrew spoken in twenty-first century Israel.

This begs a few words about the Hebrew language. Hebrew is the ancient language of the Jewish people. The Five Books of Moses, also known as the Bible or the Old Testament, are written in ancient Hebrew. Hebrew fell into disuse as a colloquial language somewhere between 200–400 CE after the majority of the Jews living in Palestine-Eretz Yisrael were forcibly exiled to Babylon. Throughout the centuries, scholars continued to write treatises and poets continued writing poetry in Hebrew. Educated Jews used Hebrew to communicate with each other regardless of where they were born and which language was spoken in their environment. Hebrew remained the liturgical language throughout the Jewish world, and children learned Hebrew through the prayer book and religious studies. Feldenkrais certainly learned Hebrew at kheyder (a kind of elementary school). In the late nineteenth century, the rise of Zionism brought about a revival of the Hebrew tongue as a spoken language. The Hebrew that Feldenkrais spoke and wrote was a product of

Hebrew's revival and the liturgical (poetic) Hebrew he had learned as a child.

Modern Israeli Hebrew is quite different from ancient Hebrew but at the same time not all that different. It is interesting to note that if an English speaker wants to read and understand a text in Old English (10th century Beowulf, for example) or a French speaker wants to read a text in Old French (11th century La Chanson de Roland, for instance) they would need to first learn Old English or Old French. Modern Hebrew speakers, even children, have no problem reading and understanding classical Hebrew writings.

Jiu-Jitsu and Self Defense, was written in literary style Hebrew that was prevalent at the beginning of the 20th century. It was more poetic than the Hebrew we speak in 21st century Israel, but I had no problem reading and understanding it. However, if I tried to speak this way, I would be accused of being pretentious. At some point, Moti asked me how I am getting along with the language. I answered that I actually had an advantage over the average Hebrew speaker because I chant Torah in the synagogue. Hence, the constructs of the language and grammar are familiar and homey to me.

When translating this book, I have attempted to retain some flavor of this very special phase of the Hebrew language. Therefore, the translation may occasionally sound a bit stilted or even ostentatious and these errors are mine alone.

— Leah Smaller

JIU-JITSU
and
SELF DEFENSE

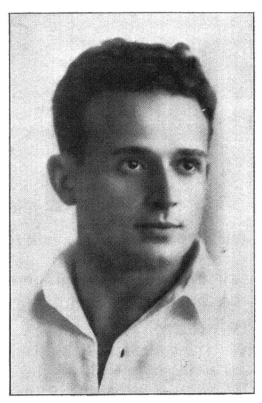

מ. פלדנקרייז

Moshe Feldenkrais

TO THE READER

The Japanese who are educated in Jiu-Jitsu do not talk about it. He does not use it except in the most extreme situations. He does not show off his knowledge.

The Japanese person who is educated in Jiu-Jitsu teaches his friends and acquaintances that which will benefit them; he teaches calmly, without causing pain, and allows himself to be bested (during practice) if only to let his comrade gain confidence in his own skills.

And you, the Hebrew reader, are asked to walk the Japanese path. However, you have a grave commitment to teach your brother the knowledge that you have acquired. Get together with a friend or two. It is easier and better to learn together. Afterward, practice with other friends; that will be my reward.

Remember, you will be stronger. To do good or evil will be in your hands. Please do not cause harm! Be careful, even with your enemies. I have gone to all this trouble and toiled at this work not in the interests of war but for Shalom (peace).

— Moshe Feldenkrais

FOREWORD

"If I am not for myself, who then is for me?"[24] An ancient saying that is still relevant today. The truth contained in this saying has helped it withstand the ravages of time.

As long as humans are on earth, there will be villains and evil men. Even the advanced civilization of our time has not winnowed out the evil and despicable from society. The civilized world is well aware of this fact and, therefore, has formulated governments, courts of law, police, prisons, and other controls. Even these institutions, which are responsible for private and public security, cannot prevent a crime before it is committed, except in exceptional cases. They usually punish the thug after he has committed his crime. But the damaged are not healed by this.

There are also worse cases than financial damage or bodily harm—and that is murder. Robbery, rape, and murder are the three malignant ills feeding on the body of society. The only immunization against them is the government. However, this immunization protects society in general and does not protect each one of us individually, in all places, at all times, and in all circumstances.

A small salvation is weaponry, whether hot or cold. The

weapon can teach good manners and abiding by laws. However, it is rightly forbidden to carry weapons because this would make it more difficult for the authorities and easier for the thugs. The regular person, the law-abiding citizen, who does not like to deal with the courts and the police is positioned between the lawbreakers, who harm his life and possessions, and the protectors of the law.

"If not the fear of the sovereign, man would eat his brother alive." And who if not the people of Israel know the truth in these words?

All nations of the world teach their sons to wield swords, shoot guns, etc. In short, they are taught to wage war. "And you protected your souls..."[25] is a commandment that all vigilantly observe, except the people of Israel. Maybe that is because of the special conditions the Jews were forced to contend with, or maybe it is because they love peace and hate bloodshed. None of this exempts them from guarding their bodies and souls. In some civilized countries, assassins are punished by death. And why should the fate of someone who allows their own lives to be taken be better than that?

Israel is vigilant regarding the laws and commandments. Guarding life is a commandment; carrying weapons is forbidden. How can a person fulfill both strictures?

Read—and you understand! Practice—and you know!

"And you teach them to your brother and your son after you"[26] and to all whose life is precious unto you.

This is compulsory, especially for police, guards, and anyone who is permitted to carry a weapon. These people risk their lives more often than someone who is not permitted to carry a weapon because danger is inherent in their occupation. If an unarmed person stumbles into a dangerous place, he will surely get out of there as fast as possible. The man who relies on his weapon may linger in such a place. A man should not rely on a machine more than he relies on his own two hands. The weapon may malfunction or be sabotaged or wrested away. Therefore, it is imperative that these people train their hands to protect their lives.

The purpose of this book is to teach every man and woman how to protect themselves with safer and more legal weapons—their own hands and limbs. The tricks and techniques that will be introduced here will help one guard his life when attacked by a multitude.

When compiling this book, I had in mind not only the muscular, strong athlete but every man, every young person whose life is precious to him and who is willing to endanger his own life to save his brother's life. With this in mind, I collected and organized the techniques and tactics from the easiest to the hardest. The first techniques described are those that do not require much practice, followed by those that require training and practice. Thus, the person who is not crazy about sports and is not interested in pursuing dexterity will immediately find what he is looking for without having to search through the pages. The young person who considers this a sport should be patient and read the first few pages, as their benefit is no less than what comes later.

I also want to apologize to the fastidious for the ruses, such as throwing sand in the eyes, which the gentle soul finds repulsive and the trained athlete will eschew. These people should understand that the goal (saving lives) is so honorable that even these means are sanctified, especially when there is no other choice.

In this book, the reader will find a selection of tactics and drills based on Jiu-Jitsu (the Japanese theory of self-defense that has gained a worldwide reputation for its excellent results). These provide a person of average or less than average strength and body size the possibility of defending himself even when faced with a stronger person armed with a club, dagger, or even a gun. In the chapter dealing with blows, the reader will find excellent blows used in boxing that one can easily learn and practice without the need of a teacher (the art of boxing itself is not acquired just by reading, but essentially requires much training). Many of the tactics in this book originate in the American wrestling style known as Catch-as-Catch-Can and those I developed through teaching and research.

Still remaining is the pleasurable task of thanking my friend Amiel Avineri (see plate 24), the founder, and coach of the Bennie Leonard Boxing Club in Tel Aviv, for his help and his participation in the majority of the photos that were taken for this book, and also to other occasional collaborators.

I am grateful to Mr. Joshua Aluf, the chairman of the national Maccabi technical board and member of the Maccabi President's Council, for reviewing all the material before it went to the printers and for his practical comments.

The reader is asked to examine the illustrations appearing in each section before he reads the section. This will save a lot of time and the text will be clearer and more understandable.

The author

Tel Aviv, 1930

INTRODUCTION

The reader who is not familiar with books of this sort may feel a great deal of discomfort while reading. However, he should remember that a savage who attacks the innocent passerby is not worthy of and does not comprehend gentle treatment. He will simply attribute it to the cowardice of the victim.

There may also be those who will say, "So, what is accomplished? After all, this [book] is practically public domain and delinquents will also read it." In fact, maybe mainly delinquents will read it, but his supposed profit will turn out to be an actual loss. First of all, to read a book and learn from it is not an easy thing for someone whose cultural level is not very developed. Secondly, people only fool themselves if they think that criminals sat idle and waited for this book to appear. It might be that they will get something out of reading these pages, but that will be negligible. They have enough of their own ruses and ploys. I will reveal here a secret known by all: the exercises and ploys in his book were actually thought up by the criminals themselves.[27]

There are those who think that the thug is a strong man with a brave heart. He is just a man like any other. He has the same courage that anyone has when attacked. Of course, some [thugs] are truly courageous, but there are also many courageous persons among [my] readers. It is worth noting that the thug's source of courage is his confidence that the victim does not know how to fight back. It is not rare to see a ruffian lose heart at the mere sight of a pistol or when serious resistance is encountered. In most instances, discovering that the victim has a weapon or that the victim puts up a firm defense will really take the wind out of his sails.

The first moment is the most important moment. The transition from an innocent passerby to an aggressive defender should occur easily, as soon as fear is put aside. To relieve the fear, breathe deeply through the nostrils with the mouth closed. Fill the lungs and expel the air little by little. Drawing a deep breath soothes the heart and quiets the heartbeat, restoring serenity and repose. It is not for nothing that we say, "take a deep breath," to signify freeing the thoughts following partial paralysis. Remember that a smile, even if it doesn't come from the heart, helps calm a person. Therefore, you should laugh lightly after drawing a deep breath, and then serenity and intelligence will replace the fear.

Paralyzing fear is not an instinctive reaction of self-preservation[28] and action expedites shedding the temporary paralysis. Many people, who are cowards by nature, do this instinctively; they perform many spasmodic gestures, such as grinding teeth, clapping hands, pulling out their hair, and suddenly transition to such a vehement attack that it is difficult to withstand. Action is the foundation of heroism and courage.

Being petrified with fear is not inherent in this person or

another and has no special virtue. It appears at the moment when a person completely stops believing in his strength and abilities, such as when an automobile is bearing down rapidly and the person sees no way to escape. The moment the frightened [person] begins to do something [to act], the paralyzing fear disappears. Therefore, he needs only to move or jump a little backward, make fists, or simply make any movement to free himself from the fear.[29] However, it is very easy to combine a deep breath with some kind of movement and then the victim will feel at least as spirited as the one attacking him.

Sometimes one needs special courage, for example, when there are rowdy goings-on at a neighbor's and he is not brave enough to endanger himself. This person should scratch his own flesh, bite his arm or lip until he draws blood. When he sees his own blood flowing, his heart fills with a valor that will later amaze him. Many people do this intuitively. The reader should not think that because he is a cultured person and the sight of blood will simply disgust him, this is not true for him; he is a human being like all others. The sight of his own blood wakes a person up and he forgets the danger. Try to remember childhood incidents and you will see that my words are true. Savages scratch their skin and make a lot of noise before they go out to confront the enemy.

When the fear has dissipated, many tricks and ruses that he reads about here will flood his memory. This is especially true if he occasionally thinks about them (*durchdenken* or "think it over to oneself.")[30] I invite the reader to think it over and he will understand that even the brave hero cannot withstand the pain in a joint, which paralyzes the heart and the consciousness.

Here I would like to point out a universal misconception. People with slight physiques, lacking bulging muscles, and whose chests are not as prominent as mountains, think that they have been less well endowed by nature compared to the bulky, strongmen. If we consider the advantages of the slighter physique (if it is not due, of course, to illness) as compared to the disadvantages of the heavier opponent, it is very difficult to decide which is preferable. The person of smaller stature need not disparage himself when confronted with the giant. The bigger and stronger a person is, the heavier and slower his movements will be. The amount of energy he expends in moving, bending, etc., causes him to tire faster than the smaller person who is quicker, more agile, and more patient. The most noteworthy advantage of a person who is tall, broad-shouldered, and more massive is his confidence in his strength, which leads him to underestimate the abilities of someone weaker than himself. When the agile, quick, and confident person (who may be weak in physical strength, but not in spirit) challenges and attacks the bulky giant, we can surmise that the victory will go to the attacker. This has been demonstrated in contests where the Japanese wrestle the European giants and also among children in the schoolyard.

The attack is no less an important means of defense as running away. When the victim begins to attack, he frees himself from fear and forces the thug to defend himself, thus diverting him from his evil intentions.

The reader will find many tricks here that are marked as dangerous. Caution must be used. The word "death" followed by exclamation points is not meant to hasten its arrival, just the opposite. The intention is to point out that, when the incident is not that serious, caution is needed when using these tactics. Remember that the goal is self-defense. The reader must keep this in mind and only use these [dangerous] ploys when there is no other choice, such as when the criminal thug is gaining the upper hand or if he is armed with a weapon, threatens life, and there is no possibility of retreat. Even in these circumstances, it is better to cause the attacker to lose consciousness or lose the ability to cause harm through some of the other ruses in this book.

Caution is especially needed during training and practice. Too strong a pull or using force beyond measure can harm the person training with you and cause him terrible injury.

Do not play around with these exercises and do not be over diligent when being observed by friends or onlookers. A person may forget himself and later be very sorry. An arm broken at the elbow, a sprained knee, a crushed throat, etc., do not heal at the same speed as they are inflicted and are never as good as before!

Important

All the tactics that appear in this book are described for one side (right or left). The symmetrical side should be practiced with the same vigor and attention.

Practicing on both sides is important not just in theory, but for practical application, too. The number of people who hold a dagger or club in their left hand is larger than would first appear. Their number is especially large amongst the benighted and ignorant who produce more criminals because right-handedness is learned at home and school.[31]

Practical Hints

During every skirmish or attack, it is important to remember that the attacker does not consider the victim's status or the victim's opinion of him. Therefore, do not explain these things to him and do not revile him. This will only annoy him and make you ridiculous in his eyes. However, a few threatening words, such as "Come any closer and I will shatter your skull" or "I'll kill the first one that moves," said in a confident tone and in a quiet voice that penetrates to the heart can sober up the attackers and also empower the one who says it.

Please remember that brute force cannot withstand pain. Poking or crushing the attacker's eye or breaking his finger or stomping on his big toe with the heel of your shoe turns even the strongest man into an innocent lamb that even a child can lead.

When you are called upon to defend yourself, do not think too much about the outcome, even if it seems that you have forgotten all the tricks you have read about here. Begin and attack; thus, your spirit will return and you will remember what you have forgotten.

- Do not talk during a fight because a sudden, wicked blow may cause you to bite your own tongue.

- Lower your head a bit. This protects your throat and eases breathing.

- Stand so your weight is more towards the toes than the heels. This stance makes it easier to transition to any movement.

- Do not strain your muscles and do not ball your fists before it is necessary. This only exhausts you and weakens your hands.

- Breathe deeply through your nose and not through your mouth.

- Do not strain your abdominal muscles because this interferes with breathing and affects your heart rate but be ready to exert them at any moment. When the abdominal muscles are relaxed, a blow to the stomach is very unpleasant and injurious.

Body Parts

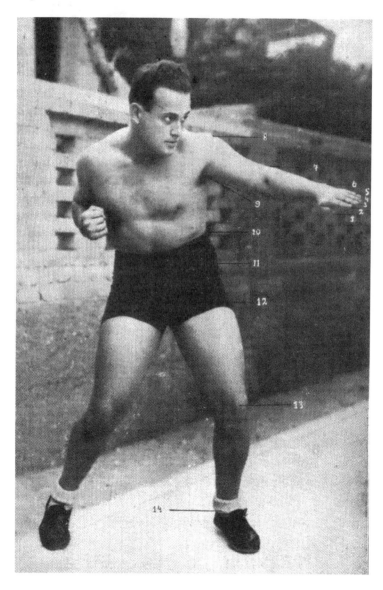

Body Part Terms

Terms for body parts are not consistent.[32] The terms used in this key to the diagram follow the usage of local sports professionals.

1. Thumb
2. Index finger
3. Middle finger
4. Ring finger
5. Pinkie
6. Wrist
7. Forearm
8. Shoulder
9. Armpit
10. Waist
11. Hip
12. Pubic bones

13. Knee
14. Ankle

5–6: Blade of the hand.
6–7: Forearm
7–8: Upper arm
12–13: Thigh
13–14: Calf

The bridge of the nose is the part of the nose that is closest to the forehead, between the eyebrows.

PART 1

Part 1 contains tricks and techniques that do not require practice or very little practice, and simply being aware of them is enough. They are meant for women and others who do not like to exercise and who do not possess great physical strength. Also included here are some tricks to use against wandering animals and animals that can cause injury.

I. Tricks to Use Against Rapists

(1) When attacked by a person who is intent on sexual molestation, there is nothing better than poking the eyes. If the attacker is hugging her in a way that leaves her arms free, she should grab his head with one hand and use the thumb of her other hand to press the corner of one of his eyes. This is extremely unpleasant, especially if it is done seriously.

(2) If only one of her arms is free, she should spread the index and middle finger, so one finger can poke one eye and the second finger pokes the other eye.

(3) If both arms are trapped or if he is holding her from behind, she should stamp forcefully with the heel of

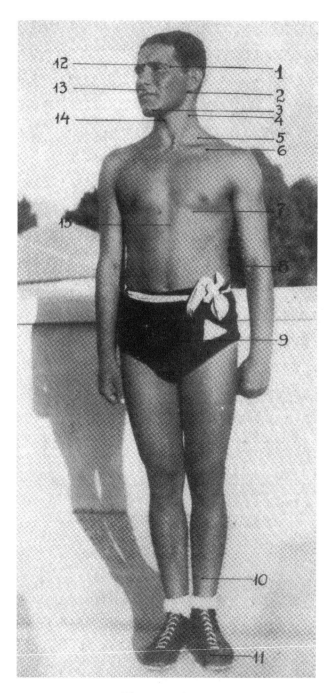

Plate 24.

her shoe on his toes in the middle of the bone below the toenail. (See plate 24, point 11).

(4) Another good tactic is stabbing his face and eyes with a hairpin. This is not very gentle, but it is wrong to behave delicately where abusiveness and brutality reign.

(5) There are rapists who cover their heads, so it is difficult to get at their eyes. In this case, it is better to put a finger in his nostril (one nostril will always be exposed for breathing) and tear it using a strong movement.

(6) Sometimes it is possible to stop the attack by simply grabbing his pinkie and bending it up towards the back of his hand, the direction that it does not bend naturally. This ploy will force the attacker to move in the direction the finger is leading him. He can be forced behind a door or forced to the ground where he can be held until help arrives.

Bending the pinkie finger can be done in two ways: a) Turn the attacker's palm up by turning the pinkie so the fingernail is facing downwards, then raise the hand holding the finger. This movement will force him to rise onto tiptoe and prevent him from taking any action. b) Twist the pinkie to turn the back of the attacker's hand up, so the fingernail is facing up, and press it down towards the floor. The rapist will be forced to bend, bringing his entire body weight forward. By pulling him forward more forcefully, it is possible to cause a head injury as he falls forward onto the edge of a table or even into a wall.

(7) A sharp blow with the toe of a shoe to the front of the shin about ten centimeters above the ankle will rob

the fearless attacker of his power. (See plate 24, point 10).

(8) When there is no other choice, a good, strong bite to the nose or ear is effective, especially if she makes an effort with her mouth; setting her teeth deep in the places mentioned and then vigorously shaking her head.

(9) Hooking a finger in the corner of the mouth and pulling strongly in the direction of the attacker's ear will also pacify him.

(10) Even though women's inner thigh muscles (adductors) are strong, it is preferable to intertwine one leg with the other. Thus, her security is increased because her grip will be stronger and she will be able to stave off fatigue longer.

(11) A woman knows how to scratch and yell, of course, so it is not necessary to mention that here. However, the attacker may put his hand over her mouth to prevent her from making a sound. Under these circumstances, if the attacker is behind her, she should grab his hands and perform the technique described in plates 48, 49, and 50. If her attacker is facing her, she should use one of the tactics described in sections 1 through 7.

II. Whatever Comes to Hand

"Whatever-comes-to-hand" is a very inclusive concept. Every object or non-object can serve as an excellent weapon against an attacker. The main thing is to know how to transform each tool or object into a weapon. Observant eyes and diligent hands can yield a benefit from anything.

(12) When an attacker is swiftly approaching or if he is on horseback, raise your left arm to protect your head from a blow with a club or whip. The body will instinctively stoop. Grab a handful of sand. Remember to pick up the sand close to the rear of your right heel. The attacker will assume that you have fallen or are afraid and he will not be aware that you have picked up sand. When he is two or three paces from you, rise up suddenly and throw the sand into his eyes. Use a fortuitous stone in the same way.

(13) A bottle full of sand or even a bottle of water can also be excellent things in an emergency.

(14) A stone, a large bolt, or even just a few silver or copper coins, or a watch tied into one corner of a handkerchief (hold the other corner in your hand) is also an excellent weapon to ward off an attacker.

(15) A bottle opener, with the sharp point protruding between your index and middle fingers and the handle held in your fist, can take the place of a dagger.

(16) Bottles filled with carbonated liquid, such as soda water, soft drinks, grape drink, kvass, mineral water thrown (after shaking well) against a wall or onto the floor can stop an angry mob and even scatter them to the four winds.

(17) When no other choice presents itself, ripping a leg off a chair or a table is easy. To do so, lift the table or chair to approximately 45 degrees. While leaning all your weight on the chair or table, a strong blow on the floor will easily snap off the leg.

(18) A large book, brought down with force, can very nicely take the place of a club.

(19) A simple glass striking on its lower edge can also confuse a person.

(20) Blows with a stick or club must be directed to the face, the base of the nose, under the ears, the mouth, the back of the neck, and the legs (between the knee and the ankle). Do not aim a blow to the top of the head or the forehead because the strongest bones are in the skull and you have to raise the club very high, which makes the movement slow.

(21) Even thin, light sticks used like spears, make excellent defensive weapons. Stabs or blows to the mouth, throat, abdomen (see plate 24 points 7, 9, 13, 14, 15) are very effective.

(22) Grab a handy chair. Spin around and, using your momentum, throw it at the attacker's legs.

(23) If the attack occurs at night in the victim's home or in a house where he is familiar with the entrances and exits, dowse the light by breaking the lamp or by some other means. The darkness will not bother the victim much, but the attacker will bump into things and fall.

(24) Any heavy tableware (heavy inkwells, spoons, etc.) are excellent missiles for self defense.

(25) When thrown horizontally, the injury caused by the edge of flat plates (used for eating meat) is more grievous than a blow with a stick, especially when it hits the face.

(26) A simple kitchen knife or a strong letter opener can become excellent daggers when stabilized using a
handkerchief that is passed between the thumb and the
index finger and then wrapped around the thumb from
above, over the index finger, around the hand and again
between the thumb and the index finger until there is no
more handkerchief to wrap. The handkerchief serves like
the handle of a dagger and protects the stabbing hand
from being cut.

(27) Sometimes a person can escape the attacker
who is threatening his life by hiding in a corridor or behind a door, which he must close behind himself. If there
is no key, it is difficult to prevent the door from opening
unless he leans his shoe (or barefoot, although this is
more dangerous) on the door, approximately 8-10 centimeters above the floor like a prop or like the supports
used for fences. He must place his leg so that the shoe is
parallel to the floor. In this manner, the door can be held
shut against the efforts of the strongest man (depending,
of course, on how strong the door itself is).

(28) If there is some object (a stick, chair, etc.)
handy, forcefully shove one end [of the stick] or the chair
legs in the gap between the floor tiles and the door. Or, if
using a chair, jam the backrest under the handle or key
if there is one. Gypsy thieves usually prop one end of a
broom against the door and stabilize the other end on the
floor using a nail if the floor is wood or putting a table or
some other heavy piece of furniture in front of the broom
if the floor is stone.

(29) All these ways of holding a door shut are useful if the door opens into the room. It is more difficult

to keep the door closed if it opens outwards, although there also many solutions; for example, a stick jammed between the handle and the door and tied with a handkerchief to prevent it from falling.

How to Stop a Fleeing Adversary

The basic difficulty in catching a malefactor is, of course, catching up with him. But that is not all there is to it. Once you have caught up with him, you must grab him and hold him so that he cannot get free and harm you. These strategies will serve you well and you will also learn to escape.

(30) First of all, the pursuer must be careful not to fall into the thug's trap. For example, he can suddenly run into a cul de sac or straight up a wall. The unsuspecting pursuer can, of course, fall prey to a blow by the thug's foot whose momentum carried him up the wall (with one foot) while he uses the other foot to vigorously kick the pursuer's belly. The scoundrel may also stop suddenly and begin to run again, causing the pursuer to lose inertia. He may suddenly turn and fall, crashing all his weight into his pursuer's chest or butt his belly or attack the pursuer's legs. All these maneuvers will harm the pursuer. The pursuer might fall backward in the first scenario, but his legs will continue moving forward through inertia. This type of fall can break a neck. In the second scenario, the pursuer's wind will be knocked out of him and a temporary paralysis will affect all his limbs. In the third scenario, he will fall forwards onto his face. All three scenarios are unpleasant and you must watch out for them.

There are indeed a number of ploys that do not endanger the pursuer and are enormously effective.

(31) Throwing a stick between the thug's legs is a good thing. Even better is grabbing his ankle with a bent-handled cane. The style of pants that feature a low, dangling crotch offers an opportune place to catch with a bent-handled cane or bent stick. You can then jerk the stick diagonally backward, pulling his feet out from under him and cause him to fall on his face.

(32) A two to three meters-long rope with some heavy object on one end can be used as a lasso. Throwing it forward and then jerking it back wraps the rope around the thug's leg (or arm), thus throwing him to the ground. (It is worthwhile practicing this on a post or a table leg.) Instead of a rope, a belt with a heavy buckle can be used.

(33) If the thug is running alongside a fence or a building, it is useful to push him into it. Through inertia, the shoulder that you push keeps moving forward and the other will hit the wall and stop. His head will be injured and he will probably fall. The collision with the wall itself will, at least, take the wind out of his sails and delay him a bit.

(34) If a punk is escaping in an automobile, there is not much to do except throw a rock in the direction of his head, especially if the rock is aimed directly at the windshield. Of course, you can also ruin the tires by shooting them out, but this option is reserved for the police or the military.

(35) A bandit on horseback can be toppled in the following manner: If the whip is in his right hand, grab

his left leg and pull him towards you and up in a plane horizontal to the horse. The spread of the horseback rider's legs is relatively small and the great pain caused by this maneuver shifts his center of gravity to the other leg and beyond. He will fall under the horse's body and between the horse's feet with one foot remaining in the stirrup. Caution!!!

(36) To stop a thug who is escaping on a bicycle: a light blow to the hand that is holding the handlebars causes the other hand to overcompensate and the front wheel will tilt horizontally relative to the road. The fall is a sure thing.

(37) Throw a stick at the frame of the bike where the legs are pedaling and not at the wheels.

Other tactics to delay fleeing scoundrels require much practice and are dangerous, so they are not within the scope of this book.

III. How to Rescue Your Brother

The maneuvers and tricks explained in this chapter are vital for people who work together and are exposed to a common danger, such as police, scouts, firefighters, and simply friends on a team. People such as these frequently need to come to the aid of a comrade who finds himself in a dangerous situation. It is possible to save a comrade from death or serious injury without putting oneself in danger by simple and direct means. Everybody can do this because all these maneuvers are as simple as can be. Quick thinking at the right time and your brother is saved and you are unscathed. Strength is not necessary for performing these maneuvers, but they should be practiced once or twice with a comrade or acquaintance.

All the maneuvers in this chapter assume that the rescuer is approaching the attacker from behind. If you are coming from the side of the victim, be careful not to call out your comrade's name because he may turn towards you. Approach as quickly as possible, push your comrade aside and take his place. You can even push him to the ground if the surface is not hard. If the attacker has a dagger or a heavy club, do not hesitate to push your friend to the ground, even if it is hard earth or a stone floor, since your comrade is not trained and you know what you are facing.

Do not forget to practice each maneuver on the right and on the left, even though the explanations are for one side only.

(38) Grab the attacker's left shoulder (either by the clothing or get hold of the shoulder itself) and use your right foot to vigorously kick the outside of the attacker's right knee. Your left hand can help the right hand (which is holding the shoulder) to spin him around, as illustrated in plate 35. After he stumbles and is falling backward, you can speed his fall by pushing with your left hand in the same direction. This trick is very easy and always succeeds. A person who falls in this manner is no longer dangerous.

(39) Encircle the attacker's neck so that your right forearm lies across his throat (Adam's apple) and your right hand is holding your own left elbow or forearm. The left hand pushes the top of the attacker's head fore-

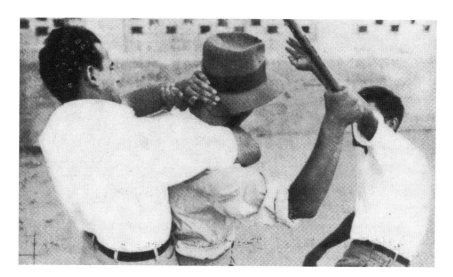

Plate 1.

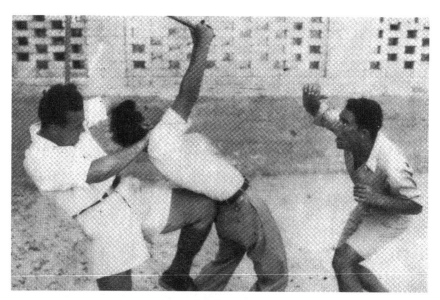

Plate 2.

word, as seen in plate 1. Now try to straighten your arms. Strangulation! Caution!!!

(40) Another excellent trick is to grab both shoulders and pull them towards you while pushing his knees, as in plate 2. As he falls, forcefully push his shoulders downwards and the impact of the fall will be greater.

(41) Grab the back of the attacker's pants as low as possible and pull him towards you and up, using your right hand to push his back forward. The pull is very painful and he will easily fall to the ground. This trick is to be used only in situations that are not very serious. You can also push the attacker forward while he is falling. His arms will come backward, and he will fall on his face. If the attacker is a heavy man, grab his pants with both hands.

(42) If the attacker is straddling your brother, who is lying on the ground, use the tactic described in section 39.

(43) Or grab the attacker's foot and pull it towards you, so his leg straightens. Now twist his foot, so his toes point to the inside, as shown in plates 3 and 4.

(44) If you arrive at the scene facing their heads [the combatants are on the ground], put your right arm under the attacker's chin and grab onto your left forearm or elbow. Your left hand should be leaning on the attacker's shoulder blade or on the back of his neck. Bend over his head, strain your arms, and try to straighten up (see plate 5). Strangulation! Caution!!!

(45) If your comrade is being attacked with a knife or club, grab the attacker's right sleeve with your right

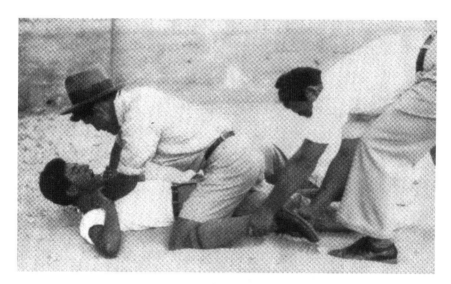

Plate 3.

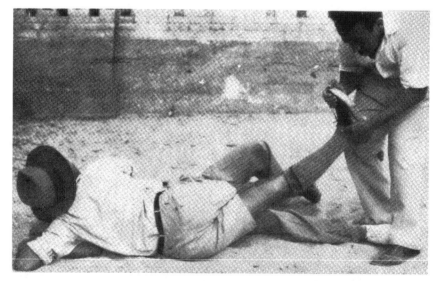

Plate 4.

hand. Place your left hand on his left shoulder and continue exactly as described in section 38.

(46) If the attacker is wielding a knife above his head, grab his hand as close as possible to his fist (even grab the fist itself) so that the back of your hand is facing down. Grab the back of his wrist with your left hand, pulling his arm down between his shoulder blades (see plate 6 and 7), and continue pulling forcefully in the direction of his heels. His shoulder will be easily dislocated (be careful!). His calves will fold under his thighs and he will fall.

This is extremely painful and prevents him from getting to his feet. This maneuver can also be done with only the right hand or with a bent-handle cane, such as a walking stick.

(47) If the attacker is strong and savage, the danger is great. It is better to pull his dagger hand backward

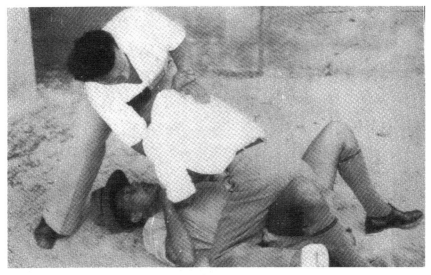

Plate 5.

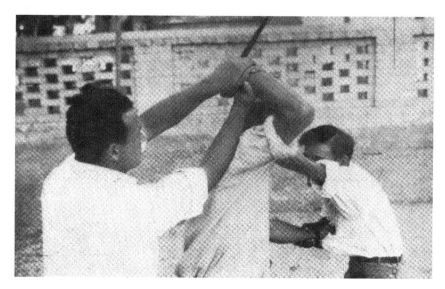

Plate 6.

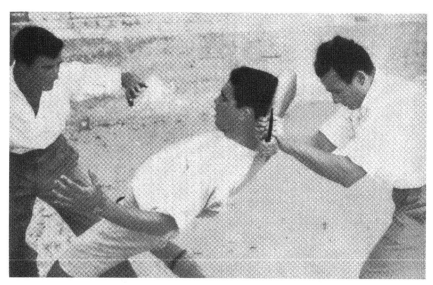

Plate 7.

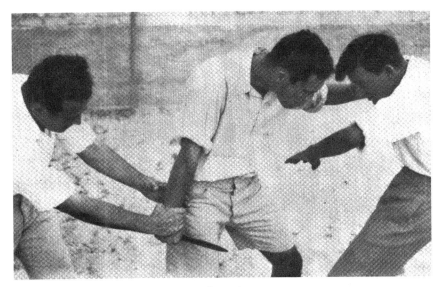

Plate 8.

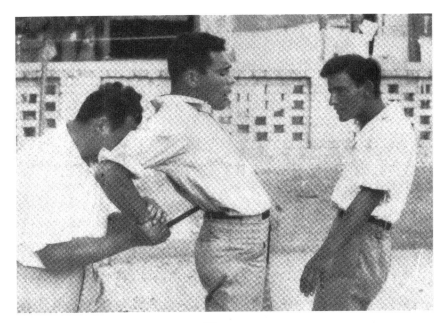

Plate 9.

and then push it forward into his own back. Caution!!! This is similar to plate 9.

(48) If the attacker is attempting to stab your comrade with an underhand knife thrust (see plate 8), it is easy to grab his hand as close as possible to his fist. Your right hand grabs from the outside and your left hand is between his hand and his body. A light, but sudden and rapid, pull backward while smashing your foot into the back of his right knee (as shown in plate 35) neutralizes the attacker.

Also, in this case, if the attacker is savage, strong, and determined in his ill intentions, you should finish the maneuver by thrusting the knife forward into his back (Caution!). The knife will injure his kidneys (see plate 9). You should avoid this tactic if at all possible.

(49) If the attacker is threatening your comrade by brandishing a club over his head, simply grab the club and pull it energetically downward. This is easy to do and is not dangerous because it is practically motionless when the club is behind the attacker's head. The result is similar to what is described in section 46 (see plates 11 and 12).

A good way to stop the club is by holding its end or middle, thus preventing its swing. Only then, grab it as illustrated in plate 11.

(50) If he is holding the club with both hands (a very common thing) and swings it sideways and up, hit him on the inside of his ankle on the weight-bearing leg in the direction of his free leg using a powerful momentum. See the place the stick is hitting his leg in plate 10.

(51) If you have a stick in your hand, hit him on his forearm approximately ten centimeters from his fist that is holding the dagger. Do not hit him on the head. Blows to the head are extremely dangerous and do not always deter the attacker. If it is impossible to hit his arm, hit his legs with great impetus about five centimeters above the ankle, at the height shown in point 10 in plate 24. If you have enough time, hit the attacker's weight-bearing leg. It is effective to hit both the arm and the legs (see plate 10).

(52) If the attacker is threatening your comrade with a gun, act according to plates 38 and 45. If you are

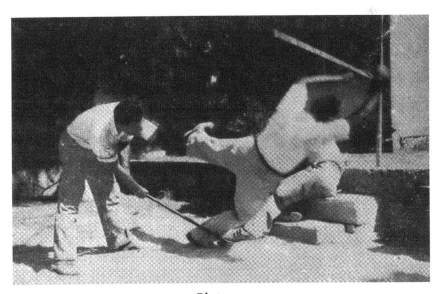

Plate 10.

holding a club, swing it and bring it down on the hand holding the gun (not on his head). The hand will drop or be deflected so it no longer poses any danger to the victim.

(53) This trick is easy. Grab the wrist of the hand holding the gun and grab the attacker's hair with your

other hand. Pull both your hands backward and, at the same time, smash into his knee as shown in plate 35.

(54) Or grab the wrist of the gun holding hand with your right hand. Quickly wrap your left hand over his arm, passing it between his arm and your right arm, and grab onto the forearm or your clothing. Plate 37 shows a similar hold done while standing in front of the attacker with the left arm under the right arm.

(55) If your comrade is attacked with a dagger stabbing up (around shoulder height) and sideways (similar to plates 36 and 46), grab the knife hand exactly as described in section 48. Jam your left shoulder into his armpit; this will turn his arm. In any case, then you can use the shoulder as leverage to use your right arm, as shown in plate 44. If there is a great difference in height between the defender and the attacker, the rescuer will pass under the arm he just grabbed (as described above) and will pull it down. Caution! The result is similar to that shown in plates 7 or 43.

(56) The attacker is straddling your comrade and brandishing a knife. Be careful not to hit him with your stick before you have kicked him (not important in which direction) because when he puts out his hand to stop his fall he can injure the victim. It is even better to kick at one of his hips and knock him onto his side.

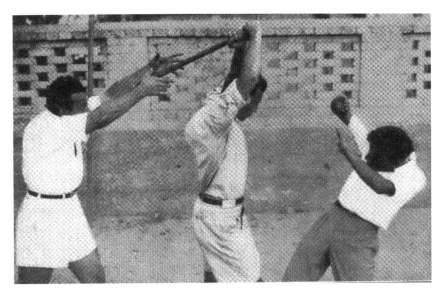

Plate 11.

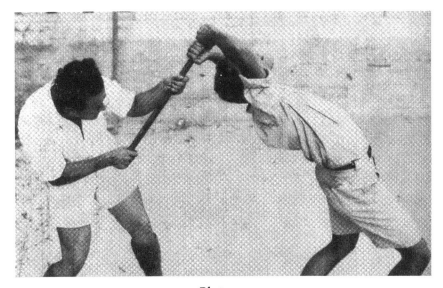

Plate 12.

IV. Defending Yourself Against Animals

The "bad" animals we may encounter in our day and age are the dog, the goat, the feral dog, and the enraged bull. Of course, we have nothing new to add about handling the street dog that barks just to bark; the best thing to do is just ignore it and keep on walking.

(a) A wolf-dog (German shepherd) is another matter altogether. Even a thick stick does not provide much protection against these dogs. It is especially important to be careful swinging the stick. These dogs have excellent senses and, calculating the moment when the stick is moving away from them, and they leap at you. It is better to wait for the dog's leap and use the end of the stick to poke him in the face or between the ribs. Sometimes a swift kick in the teeth is also successful.

(b) If attacked by a dog in a village or outside a city, where there are not many people, it is best to sit down on the ground and pivot, so you are facing the dog. In this situation, you can use the stick to injure the dog's legs. Although the dog would certainly attack a man standing and brandishing a stick, experience has shown that no dog will dare to attack a human being in this position. If you do not have a stick, it is helpful to crawl on all fours, like an animal, with a handkerchief or hat in your mouth or on your head. Even the most daring dog does not attack a man crawling and growling. When the dog starts barking, move your legs in all sorts of ways and make strange noises. A dog will not come too near a person doing this.

(c) If a dog has jumped you and is holding you by the throat, you have no choice but to crush his eyes. Dogs do not attack with one bite, like wolves, but with a series of deep bites. There is enough time to poke his eyes and a strong person can sometimes succeed in choking the dog.

(d) Quickly get out of the way of a stray dog foaming at the mouth. Throwing sand in its eyes is very useful, but the dog will continue to attack. Take off your coat or some other piece of clothing and wave it in front of you. The dog will bite the coat and not let go. Tease the dog by trying to wrest the coat away. This will allow you to get to a door or a big rock. Be careful! Do this quietly and reasonably.

(e) The bull is already moving and is enraged at seeing something red. If it has begun to run towards you, throw the red object or clothing onto the ground and, when the bull is five to six meters away, slip past him and run in the direction from which he is coming. The bull is incapable of stopping suddenly and it will take some time to turn. If there is no other retreat, this tactic will wear out even the strongest bull. When dealing with a stray cow, you must be more careful because she is lighter and quicker than a bull. Let the cow get much closer, two to three meters. This is very dangerous.

V. Miscellaneous

In the preceding chapters, we saw how it is possible to rescue someone from an attacker. All the tricks presented were really quite serious as a person's life is dependent upon the results. In this chapter, we will present a few useful ruses to separate combatants and enemies.

To separate two people in a clinch, put your hands on their faces with your fingers spread like *Birkat Ha'Kohanim* (Priestly Blessing).[33] Your forearms will press under their noses. Pushing your hands outwards will separate the combatants easily. Plates 20 and 65 show this hand movement.

(57) It is easy to separate two combatants by putting the blade of your hand on their throats and pushing them aside. Be careful not to go overboard with this movement, so you don't damage their throats.

(58) If the adversaries are holding on to each other's clothing, it is useless to grab a hand and try to pry it loose. This will only be an annoyance and give the other one an opportunity to take control of his rival. In this case, it is best to come between them aggressively. If this is difficult, raise both your arms and bring them down forcefully on their arms. Then, step between them.

(59) If one adversary is much stronger than his opponent and his attack is extremely savage, throw your coat over his head and face. By the time he extricates himself, his opponent will have taken the opportunity to get far away.

(60) It is useful and very easy to grab the coat of one of the combatants (if it is not buttoned) and raise it as far as possible above his head. It is difficult for him to free himself and it is possible to hold someone like this until he calms down.

(61) It is also possible to pull the coat down, trapping the attacker's arms. Grab the edges of the collar, or lower, from both sides. Open the coat, dragging it down to the middle of the arms; this forces his hands together.

His arms are trapped with no way out. It is easy to do this from in front as well as from the rear.

(62) To stop someone who is running away, it is useful to throw a piece of clothing, a blanket, or any similar object over his head.

(63) If the stronger attacker is wearing a fedora, grab the front of the brim in one hand and put your other hand on the back of his neck. The head and the hat are not round but a bit elongated, which gives you double leverage. Rotate the hat turns his head. After turning his head aside, you can drop him to the ground by pulling the hat down. It is important to drag the hat brim down while turning it.

(64) If he is wearing a soft cap, grab the visor and pull it over his nose. The hat will block his view. He will surely try to free himself and the victim will have time to get away.

(65) Sometimes it is necessary to remove a pest or a drunk. Grab his head between your hands so that one hand is behind his head and the other hand is pressing under his nose with the knuckles pressing against his mouth. The knuckles prevent him from breathing through his mouth and the hand under his nose blocks his nostrils. This, together with the pain that is causing his eyes to tear, allows you to press your hands towards each other and force him to stand.

(66) It may happen that when hurrying to summon a doctor from someplace of entertainment or on some other mission that cannot be delayed, he finds his way blocked by a crowd in a narrow passageway. If he

tries to force his way through, he will anger the people and also pointlessly exhaust himself. It is better to squat down and make your way among the crowd's legs. There is a lot more space at this height than when standing erect, where chests and shoulders fill the whole space.

(67) Urgency may justify the following. Boost yourself onto an elevated area, such as a window ledge or some other protuberance, or even up onto the shoulders of people on either side of you. Continue on your way, walking on the crowd's heads and shoulders. Obviously, this cannot be done every "Montik and Donershtag"34 (a Yiddish expression meaning "routinely.") First of all, it is not ethical, and second, those responsible for maintaining public order will most certainly punish you for it. In exceptional circumstances, when a person's life is at stake or when someone is depending on you, do not hesitate: get up and go. A bit of courage and sharp sightedness will serve you well. Do not be afraid. In places where "a needle cannot fall to the ground," a person will also not fall.

PART 2

Introduction

This chapter contains tricks and ploys that are generally used in Jiu-Jitsu and Catch-as-Catch-Can. All these tricks require training. Brute strength is ineffectual here; however, sudden and swift exertion is required. Thus, relaxation and exertion should be practiced. Relaxation increases patience and eliminates fatigue so that power is available for active exertion.

The entire body should be trained at relaxation and exertion, each limb separately and together. It is good to learn to exert the hands without exerting the abdominal muscles; this way breathing doesn't stop during the action.

The method of relaxation and exertion is very important, but the space here is too limited to go into details. Thus, it is a good idea for the reader to watch a cat fighting a dog (or another cat) and observe how all its muscles are relaxed until the last instance when it exerts them as quick as lighting as if struck by an electrical current.

It is [also] a good idea for the reader to watch a boxing lesson given by an expert or visit a professional dancing studio to see exactly how it is done. Relaxation is not so crucial that these tricks cannot be done without it, but much more can be achieved with its aid than without it.

The tricks in this section include many that will amaze the reader and will seem impossible. For example, plates 23, 29, 33, 43, 56, and 60.

How is this done? Is his left hand free and he can hit me with it? Or is he holding a stick, which he can use to shatter my skull, in his other hand? Several examples will clarify this. All living beings cannot shift their attention from a painful spot. Pain is paralyzing and can cause loss of consciousness. For clarity, I will use an example, which the wise reader will excuse me for using.

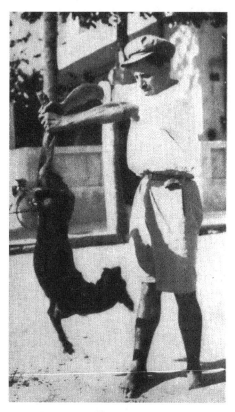

Plate 13.

When catching a man by his privates, he will do nothing but grab the hand holding him. How could he grab his attacker's throat? The pain is so great that he cannot think of anything else. All attention is directed to the painful area and he cannot see or think of anything else.

Not only does man be- have in such a way, but

also other living beings. For example, the dog in plate 13 is vigorously trying to grab and sink his teeth into the hand holding his leg. He is exhausting himself to no avail since he cannot reach it. His teeth are so close to the thigh of his captor, why not sink his teeth into that? He can see it, but his attention is not directed to it; his attention is on one thing—his leg! The pain and fear nail his attention to the trapped leg, just like a man grabs the hand that is causing him pain and ignores everything else.

When a person makes a movement or executes an action that demands his attention, he will continue his action or movement even if he is suddenly and momentarily delayed. For example, in tricks 48 and 49, the attacker could have easily absconded unharmed if he would have let go of the stick he was brandishing as soon as he felt another person's hand grabbing him. Yet, he will not do so. On the contrary, he will hold it [the stick] more forcefully. Technique 48 shows how it is possible to divert the hand holding the dagger, so the attacker drives the knife into himself through his determination to continue the movement he initiated. Your action only increases his desire to follow through with the movement he has begun.

There will be those who will say, "How can a man in mortal danger remember a complex trick or ploy and how will he know which trick to use at that moment?" This is a good question. However, the reader should keep in mind that using a gun is much more complicated and difficult than using the hands, and yet, don't people benefit from using it? A gun should be used only when in grave danger. The principle is training; the trained person can do anything. The reader who closely examines all the tricks in this book will realize that each one begins with the instinctive movements a person makes when he is attacked in the manner described. Anyone who sees a dagger raised to strike at his head will protect it [his head] with one of his hands, even if he has not heard of or read this book. On the other hand, if he is the one brandishing a stick or knife to strike another person on the head, he will see that person raise his hand to protect himself as in plates 2, 25, 27, 36, and so on.

Experience shows that the moment a person under attack feels the touch of the aggressor's body on one of his limbs, he is freed from his momentary paralysis. He then performs the whole maneuver with the same ease as in training, perhaps even better.

Techniques 83-95 should actually be regarded as one; if the defender happened to extend his right [hand] first, he would proceed like this, and if he extends his left hand first, he will proceed in such a way. Therefore, the defender doesn't have to determine how to react before he actually begins. The reaction comes by itself, instinctively. Thus, the techniques become as simple as can be.

Notice that all strategies are designed for the situation of the aggressor holding a weapon while the defender has nothing [no weapon] at all. The attacker doesn't consider the possibility of any sort of defense, so of course, he isn't careful and doesn't try to outsmart his victim. Instead attacks him furiously without assessing the situation. These techniques are to be used only in circumstances where the attacker's intention is not entertainment but rather murder and rape.

The sparring partner should imagine that he is acting in the aforementioned circumstances.

The novice should pay attention to this. A trained person will easily overcome even this difficulty. But not so the beginner, who wishes to show off to his friends or acquaintances.

Training with partners should be done on a mat or soft sand. When the attacker's hand touches the defender, the former must immediately release his friend because all sorts of muscle damage can occur, such as inflammation, stretching, etc., sometimes even spraining and breaking bones.

Act quickly and energetically, but don't be [too] enthusiastic. Don't forget that over-zealousness often ends in sorrow.

Whoever wants to learn these tricks must maintain and develop his body's health, agility, and patience. Here are some precepts and prohibitions that should be observed:

- Don't eat to satiation.
- Don't eat more than three times a day. A full stomach is badly injured even with the slightest stab. A full stomach makes you slow, makes your movement heavy, interferes with your breathing, exhausts your strength, and tires the heart.
- Chew your food very well.
- Don't drink during a meal. Food that has been chewed well mixes with saliva and becomes a slippery compound that is easily swallowed.
- Run about 1000–1500 meters once a week.
- Go to bed early.

If you observe these [precepts], you will defend yourself more ably than if you workout every day but don't observe them.

The strength of the fingers, palm, and forearm is important for all the techniques in this book. He who trains his body for self-defense should know that even if he has a strongman's arm but a weak hand, his hold will have no effect on his rival beyond the strength of his hand. Most sportspeople, especially track and field athletes, train all their muscles and ridiculously neglect the hand's palm, finger's muscles, and the muscles of the balls of the feet and toes. This is not true for the Jiu-Jitsu trainee, the boxer, and fencing student.

The Japanese people increase the strength of their palms and fingers by squeezing a packet of paper, transferring it from one hand to the other, turning and squeezing until it is compacted. They then add more paper, so the packet is big enough for the fingertips to participate in the squeezing. This kind of squeezing and hand movement in all directions, with a fist and with straight fingers, very quickly increases the strength of the hand. When the hand tires out, it should be raised over the head and shaken for a moment until it is completely relaxed, and the fatigue will instantly pass.

Practical Instructions

Don't decide in advance, "this technique would help me." Learn them all and use the ones that most suit your spirit and build on those that you know better.

Don't use cunning ploys in your defense against an untrained person, as he will not comprehend the finesse of your actions and you will only lose.

Be careful not to bloody your attacker because it will energize him. The people around you will take his side, and it's punishable by law.

Look the attacker in the eyes; there, you will see all his apparent and hidden intentions. There are boxers who look only at their opponent's feet, which is a very good thing to do, as the opponent cannot see your eyes. However, this requires much practice and a sharp and perceptive eye.

Don't call out for the police for help if you are attacked in an isolated corner. The aggressor knows better than you do where the police officer is at that time. Thugs always have a good enough reason to not come face to face with a policeman and by calling out, you will force your attacker to silence you with his knife or his gun, while all he meant was only, perhaps, to rob you. When walking a woman home in the dark, don't pay attention to any catcalls at your or her expense unless it is impossible to ignore. Swiftly and without hesitation, use one of the blows shown in this section. Then, without further ado, continue on your way quietly and safely. It will take the wind out of the interloper.

If you see suspicious persons approaching you, be prepared! If they are not concealing their evil intentions, be the first to attack! If you attack first, you will have the advantage.

Do not fear the number of attackers. Remember that two are more dangerous than ten. Ten cannot catch one [person] at the same time. They get in each other's way.

Do not forget to run away at the right moment. The English say that the one who fights and runs away lives to fight another day.[35] I didn't suggest this practical instruction in the first part because I assumed that it is obvious. Although the young athlete might think it is a shame to run away, this is not so! Even Achilles ran away. A coward runs away from a fight before doing what he should have done; the fond of life run for dear life after risking that life!

Do each trick as quickly as you can but not hastily. Haste is not speed!

VI. The Fall

The fall is one of the most important things for protecting yourself in a brawl. The attacker will always try throwing his victim to the ground if he has not succeeded in harming him while standing. In this situation [lying on the ground], it is much harder for an untrained person to extricate himself and then running away is not possible. For these reasons, brawlers try to knock each other down.

However, the man that knows how to fall not only avoids being injured by the fall but uses the fall to aid in distancing himself from his attacker. With the correct fall, he moves away from the spot where he was standing by lowering himself but stays on his feet, much to the attacker's surprise.

You must practice falling forward and backward as the benefits of a good fall are many (I myself was saved from twice death thanks to knowing how to fall). This is important not just in a brawl but in a person's daily life as well.

One who knows how to fall correctly can use the fall as an excellent strategy. He will not injure himself if he intentionally falls while holding on to the attacker, whereas the one taken along in the fall will be severely injured.

The plates illustrating the correct forward and backward falls were intentionally taken without too many garments, on a stone floor, and with hard-soled shoes (not sports shoes) to show that a correct fall doesn't even scratch the skin and that street shoes are not a hindrance. In the forward fall, one hand touches the ground while the other arm protects the head, which is bent towards the chest as much as possible.

The right knee is bent when the left arm is protecting the head and vice versa (the plate illustrates the second case). Even falling at medium speed, the impetus brings a person to his feet. Come to standing on one foot as described in plate 16, as this is much easier. If the impetus is very slow, come to standing by helping with the hand that touches the ground first (same plate).

When falling backward, bring the head strongly towards the chest because if you don't, it will smash on the ground. It is important, as well, to fall with the largest possible area

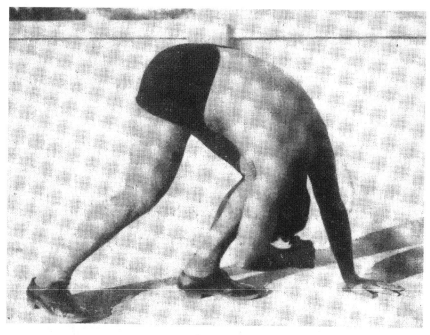

Plate 14.

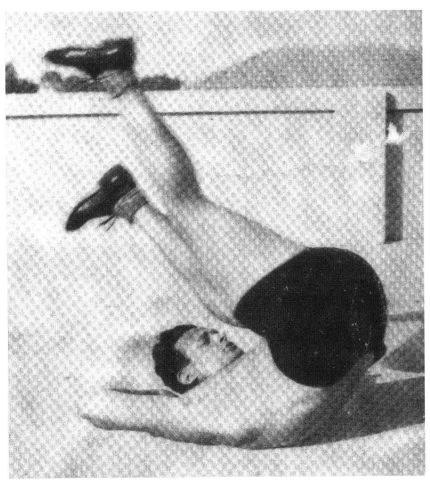

Plate 15.

of the body hitting the ground at the same time and not land on places and points that stick out, like the backside or elbows. These protrusions suffer during a fall. Be careful to keep the arms rigid and let the shoulders touch the ground (as illustrated in plate 17). When the area touching the ground is large, the impact of the fall is weakened. Although there are those who recommend getting up from this fall with the head lowered to one shoulder, experience shows that the approach described in plate 18 is easier and

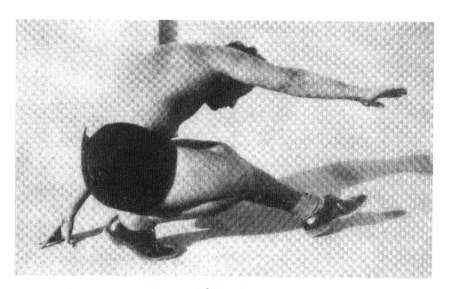

Plate 16.

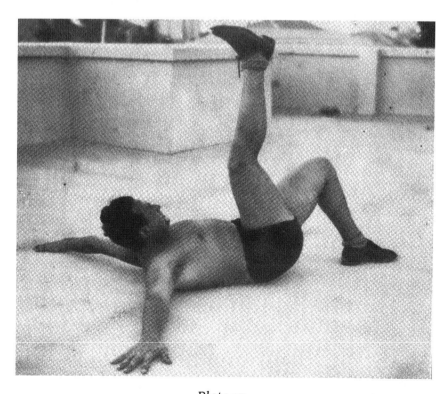

Plate 17.

also better. This is especially true when the ground is not level—falling over a curbstone, for example. If his hands do not touch the ground first, then a person falls with his entire weight on his nape.

Falling to the side is more relevant to sports and will not be described here. However, it is worth keeping in mind that an arm outstretched towards the ear and straight at the elbow will not be damaged during the fall and will also decrease the impact. See plate 10. The person falling extends his arm upwards and falls correctly.

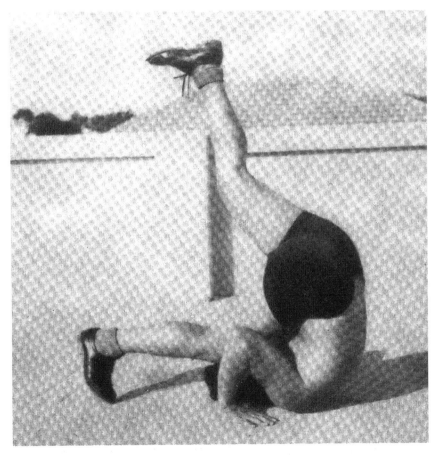

Plate 18.

Being tripped is not dangerous to a person who has learned how to fall well both forward and backward.

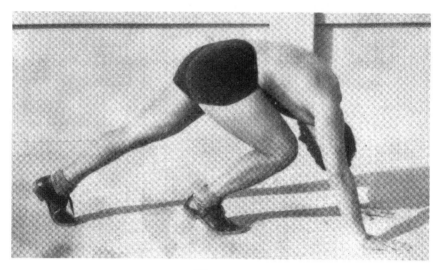

Plate 19.

VII. Throws and Tripping

To topple a person, try to hold as close as possible to the tips of his fingers and toes. These places, farthest from the center of the body, are weaker and can be hurt more easily. Their distance from the center of gravity enables using them as leverage.

(68) In plate 20, the defender spreads his hands as much as possible and pushes, using a sawing motion. One hand placed under the nose pushes the head down and back, while the other hand helps by grabbing the attacker's thigh and flipping him face down. This is the longest lever available in this situation.

(69) Positioning the legs is an important detail.

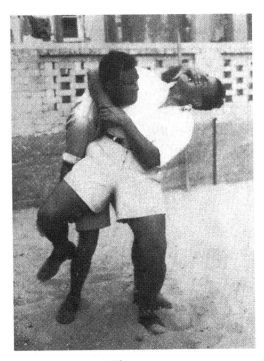

Plate 20.

Plate 21 shows how to position the legs correctly. Position a leg behind both legs of the person wielding the club and then quickly sink to one knee. The hand on the side of the kneeling leg is ready to lean on the ground and the other hand helps the obstructive leg, thus causing the attacker's knee to fail. The attacker is trapped between the leg and the arm as if between the blades of dull scissors that, although they do not cut paper, topple him over.

The arm must be very straight at the elbow and the knee must be facing forward, so the attacker's fall does not break your leg. You bend and turn to kneel on the ground.

(70) You can position the leg so that the attacker falls on his face and not backward. The movement is similar to what is described above. However, the defender must turn himself in the same direction the attacker is facing.

(71) It is easier and less dangerous to throw the attacker, as described in plate 22. Lowering his head, the defender takes a very large step forward and stoops to-

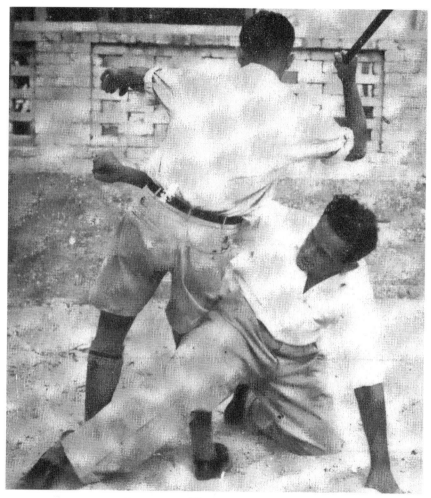

Plate 21.

wards the ground to grab the attacker's heel with both hands (see plate). He pulls the heel powerfully toward his chest while pressing his shoulder into the attacker's calf. A simple fall will be enough to take the wind out of the assailant's sails on a stone floor or the street. On sand or soft earth, you can finish off with the [technique] illustrated in plate 23. The handhold should be familiar and is shown clearly in the picture. The tendons in the ankle

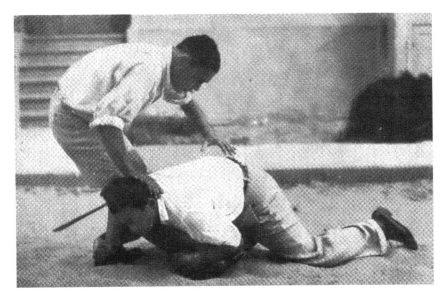

Plate 22.

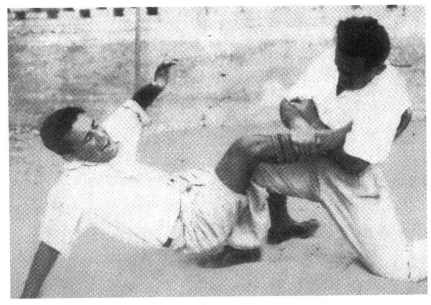

Plate 23.

are stretched beyond their limit by the defender's body, which is leaning backward and pressing one hand down and the other hand up.

Remember! If the assailant is much stronger than the defender, who is supine on the ground, it is better to stay down than to get to his feet. When confronting a stronger and heavier opponent, there is no better, more comfortable, and more secure position than lying on the ground. Clearly, we are not talking about an assailant who is holding a gun or a heavy club, but rather a strong man who simply uses his physical strength. If you are standing, your opponent's weight will topple you to the ground and his blows are heavy as well. Lying on the ground, the difference in weight is not that important and the assailant must fend off not only the fists of the person on the ground but also his legs. Blows by the legs, especially of a light person, are heavier than those of his fists. In addition, trick 95 will rescue you from dire straits.

(72) It is very easy to throw a person to the ground using the technique illustrated in plate 43 and described in detail in section 92. Otherwise, simply grab one of his [the assailant's] hands with both of your hands, pull it forcefully towards yourself, so you straighten up. Then lift it quickly above your head and pass under it to the most comfortable side. Try this with a friend. Practice it to both sides, turning once to the right and once to the left. Do this very, very slowly, so you do not endanger your hand. Find the most suitable direction for your body structure and practice this trick turning to your comfortable side.

VIII. Blows and How to Defend Yourself from Them

There are three types of blows done with the hands: 1: Blows with fists, a method of attack and defense, which is the science of boxing. 2: Blows with the edge of an open and flat hand, where the continuation of the pinkie makes contact (this maneuver is called *Handkante-schläge*,[36] in German). 3: Finger stabbing.

1. Blows with the Fists

A punch must be delivered with a nicely formed fist, where the thumb lies over the other fingers! You will sprain your thumb if it is tucked inside. The joint connecting the hand and the third finger must be the one that connects with the target when striking the blow (see plate 25). The fist must be in line with the forearm, so it is very firm and will not bend to either side. The blow must be as rapid as possible, travel the shortest distance, and use the body's full weight. As the Englishman says, punching begins from the toes. Indeed, this wallop has value.

(73) The best and hardest blow that the fist delivers is illustrated in plate 25. A fast, sharp blow to this spot [the chin] will knock your opponent out of the fray. In boxing terminology, this is called a K.O. (Knock Out), and the spot is point 3 in plate 24. It can be delivered from the other side as well.

(74) The second [type of blow] is not less effective than the first and is easier to use against a tall aggressor.

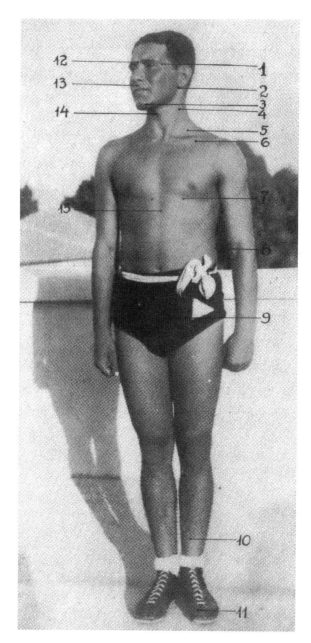

Plate 24.

It is delivered to the solar plexus, the point labeled 15 in the same plate 24. A sudden whack at this place robs the aggressor of the possibility of moving or making a sound for several seconds. Blows to points 1, 2, 7, 12, 13, and 15 are also severe. How can you protect yourself from these blows?

The best way is to jerk aside; even a small step that tilts the body sideways is enough. The person, intending to land a harmful blow, will strike at air and momentarily lose his balance. You can take advantage of this to hit him using any of the blows described here or kick his knee as shown in plate 35, or trip him, and so on.

2. Flat Handed Blows

(75) A trained, formidable hand is a very danger-ous weapon. One must be cautious and use it only in extreme situations. These blows should be delivered to the places described in plate 24, points 2, 4, 5, 6, 9, 8, 13, 14, 15. These spots are very sensitive and a blow at these points causes great damage. These places should be avoided whenever possible. Extra care should be taken with blows to spot 14. Even the lightest blow in this spot will disable a person. A rapid blow here can even cause death! Caution!!!

[Blows to] the spots marked 2 and 4 and the back of the neck (not shown in the picture) are also very dangerous.

Flat-handed blows must be delivered with the palm and forearm in a straight line, so at the moment of contact, the arm and forearm are, if possible, at right angles to the elbow. The hand should not pause at the point of

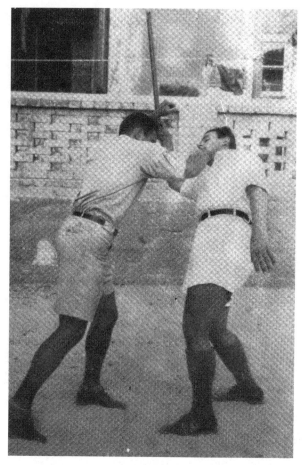

Plate 25.

contact because the blow should be quick with a springy recoil. The back of the hand should be facing upwards, as illustrated in plate 26.

The edge of the hand must be hardened through training. At first, try hitting your own knee; later, you can use a sack filled with sand or sawdust, moving on to smooth wood, rough wood, smooth stone, walls, and finally, rough stone. You can achieve this with only one minute of training a day for the first few weeks. This

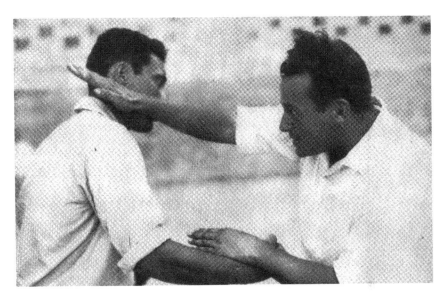

Plate 26.

type of blow is equal to a clout with a thick, strong club. After a few weeks of training, a blow with the edge of the hand (even in the places marked 6, 8, and 9) may prevent the aggressor from continuing his attack. However, it is better for the defender to choose one of the other techniques, which are less life-threatening to the aggressor.

Of course, a hand that has been hardened in this way can be used as a defense against the same type of blow and also against blows from a club. It is also easy to defend yourself from this type of blow using the techniques shown in plates 22 and 23.

When the hand is unformed and soft, it is better to use the fists. However, in a very short time and with very little effort, it is possible to turn the edge of the hand into an inconspicuous weapon, a weapon that is always close by and tested, always handy. Boxing is much harder to learn.

3.   Stabbing with the Fingers

Stabbing with the fingers is within the scope of this book. Although the Japanese do wonders with it, striking their target exactly with their hardened and trained fingertips. The timing and cool head required make it ineffective as a defensive measure. The only stabbing action that should be mentioned here is poking a finger in the eye.

Defensive techniques against simple blows are exactly the same as those used against knife attacks. Simple blows are clearly less dangerous; therefore, you can defend yourself against them with ruses that are less energetic and less drastic.

(76) Like the attack shown in plate 36, a raised fist can be stopped, as illustrated there. Otherwise, turning your body towards the attacker's right, grab your hand as illustrated in plate 60. You can cause him more pain if you hold your right hand not on his chest but on his shoulder joint.

(77) When the attacker is much taller than you, it is better to finish off by wrapping your left hand under his elbow and grabbing your right hand, which is holding the attacker's upper arm, or grabbing his arm as shown in the picture (see plates 55, 56, and 60). Now straighten your elbows. If you bear down a little, you can break the attacker's arm at the elbow (see also plates 36 and 37).

(78) To defend yourself against an assailant who is raising his right fist to strike you from the side (as in plate 34), use your right hand to stop his swing as illustrated there and finish as described in section 31 (see plate 35).

(79) You can defend yourself against a fist raised to strike you in the head, as described in chapter 10 (plates 27–33). Study chapter 10 "Defending Yourself Against a Club and a Dagger."

(80) To defend yourself against various blows, you can use the tactic of throwing your opponent to the ground, as described in the chapter Falls and Tripping. (See sections 68–72 and plates 21, 22, and 23.)

(81) In the East, they often use the head to strike blows. Defend yourself against head blows to the stomach by smashing the [attacker's] head on your knee. Increase the force by positioning your hands on the crown of his head and giving a tremendous push. (See plate 26a).

(82) [If the aggressor] is using his head to strike at your face, lift your elbow; his face will suffer much. An effective remedy for a fist straight to the face is described in section 80 or use one of the boxing punches.

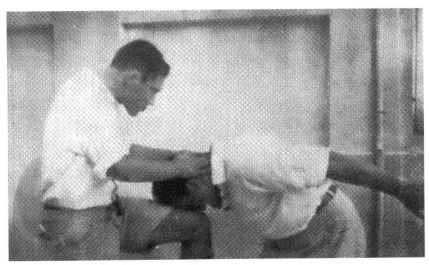

Plate 26a.

IX. Defending Yourself Against a Club and a Dagger

When defending yourself against a man wielding a club, first of all, remember that it is impossible to bash someone with a club when the target is standing too close. Secondly, if the swing is very powerful, then the oscillation will be long (according to the laws of nature). Thirdly, the strength of the club's blow increases from the fist [holding the club] to the point known in physics as the "point of oscillation" and then again decreases. From this, we learn that it is necessary to be as close as possible to the one holding the club because, in this situation, the club becomes a hindrance.

It is possible to spring towards the blow at the apex of the upswing or at its beginning (see plate 25). It is imperative to stop the club as close as possible to the hand that is wielding it (same plate).

Obviously, the point is to train the eye and practice the timing for the leap forward. You can learn to judge the correct moment to leap quite well after a few days of easy training and some simple exercises. Illustrations that detail this may make it appear complicated and difficult. It is better to learn from experience. Study well what is written here, give the club to a good friend, and let him hit you. Start slowly, slowly until you learn to get close to him as he strikes a blow.

Important! If the attacker is waving the club from side to side, lift your elbows high when you leap towards him. A blow to the wrist is worse than a blow to the hips or torso because it prevents you from continuing to defend yourself.

Use the edge of the hand to stop the club's swing, as in the photos illustrating defense against a knife attack. It is better to allow the strike to come down on the forearm rather than any other spot that is raised to protect the head (see plates 25 and 27).

In addition to the tactics for defense against a knife attack, the techniques against being cudgeled from above (described in plates 21, 22, 23, and 25) and the tricks shown in (plates 34, 35, 36, 37) and those described in sections 76–78 are useful.

The following two tricks are also useful:

(a)   As soon as the attacker raises the club to strike you, lower your head to your chest and, with a quick movement (running or leaping), bring it under the armpit of the [aggressor's] raised arm or, at least, to the side of the body with the raised arm. While leaping, make a fist, grab the fisted hand's wrist, turn it so the elbow leads and strikes the attacker. The leap itself and the forward movement of both arms position the elbow to forcefully strike the attacker's solar plexus[37] (point 15 in plate 24). This will easily topple him to the ground in a state of partial paralysis and semi-consciousness. If the attacker is holding the club in his right hand, lift your right elbow and vice versa; lift the left elbow if he is holding the club in his left hand.

(b)   As soon as the attacker lifts the club in his right hand, for example, quickly bend over and bring your right hand and your entire upper body under his raised

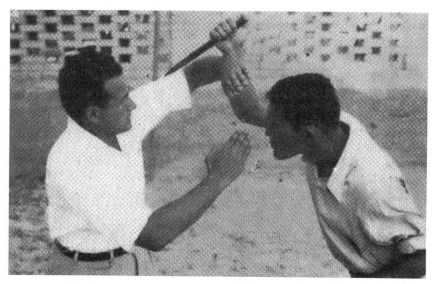

Plate 27.

arm. Straighten your elbow, place your right hand on his hip or on his torso, and push him forward. Your right leg, positioned in front of his leg, prevents him from stepping forward. The hand pushing him transfers the center of gravity forward, forcing him to fall on his face. All these movements must be done quickly, as one whole movement. The fall occurs because the conditions created are similar to those described in the movement resembling the paper and dull scissors (see the introduction to this section).

Defending yourself against a dagger attack is most dangerous. First of all, the assailant armed with a dagger or knife means to murder and he will be very savage. Secondly, a blow from a knife is fatal and causes more damage than a club. With this said, defending yourself is relatively easy from a technical standpoint. The person armed with a knife who attacks a person standing empty-handed is so sure of his prey that he does not really consider the possibility of opposition. For clarification, study the introduction to this chapter.

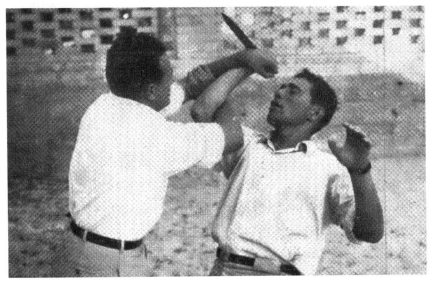

Plate 28.

The four main stabbing styles are described in plates 27, 34, 36, and 38. As we already mentioned in the introduction, each type can be opposed in two ways: by extending and lifting the right hand or the left hand. The plates are adequate and further explanation is superfluous.

(83) When the attacker is wielding a dagger over your head, and your first movement was with your left hand, defend yourself as described in plates 27, 28, 29, 30.

Accustom yourself to extend the defensive arm with the elbow bent at 90-degrees. If the elbow is not bent at 90 degrees, the attacker's hand can slide along your arm and injure you.

You can finish this off a bit differently: after your left

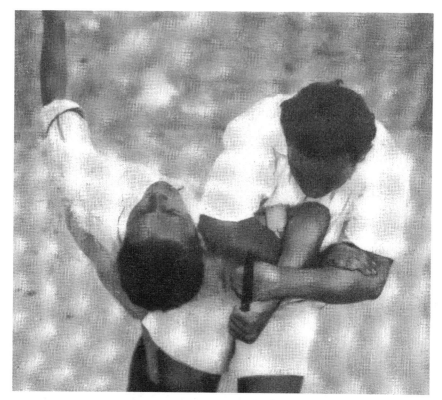

Plate 29.

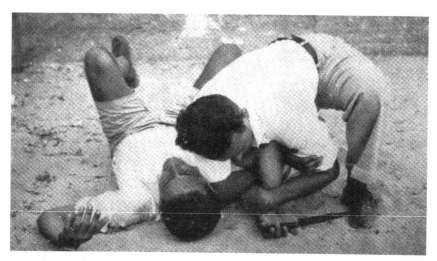

Plate 30.

hand has delayed the hand brandishing the dagger, lift your right hand so that the attacking arm is placed on the elbow and grab the front of the left hand, which is balled into a fist. Now connect the elbows and squeeze the hand that is lying between your hands. The finish can be as shown in plate 30 or plates 30, 31, 32, and 33.

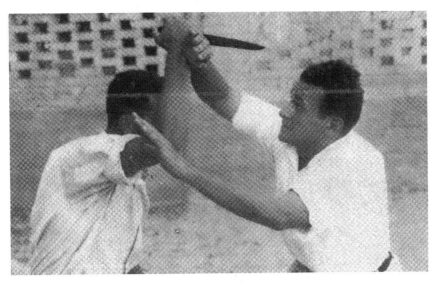

Plate 31.

If the first [movement] was with the right hand, pay attention to strike the attacker's elbow with your left, as shown in plate 32. The protective hand should be far enough away from the head or neck so the blade will not harm you even after you stopped the hand from delivering the blow. Study plates 27 and 31 well. The protective arm is bent at the elbow, extending forward as far as possible, and the head is moving backward.

(84) If your life is threatened by an assassin who is stabbing forward, reach out with your right hand as in plate 34, defend yourself as shown in plate 35 (see section 38). After your right hand has blocked the dagger's

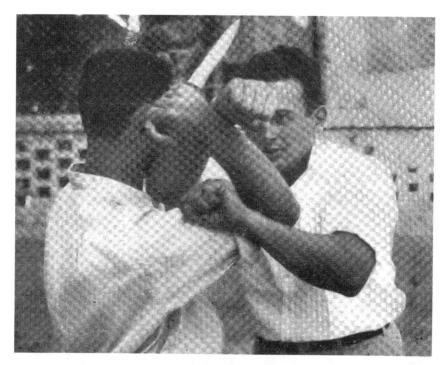

Plate 32.

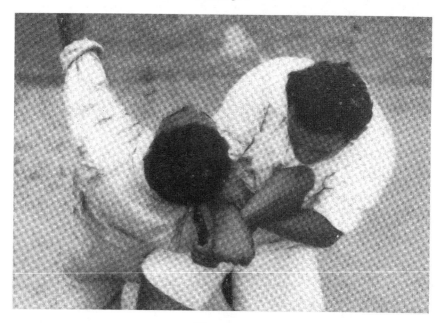

Plate 33.

swing, use your other hand to grab the assailant's clothes near the attacking arm's shoulder and push forward. Simultaneously move your left leg in front of his right leg and kick it backward forcefully. Your arm and leg, moving opposite one another, topple him. Your push forces the aggressor to transfer all of his weight onto the leg that you have kicked and he will surely fall.

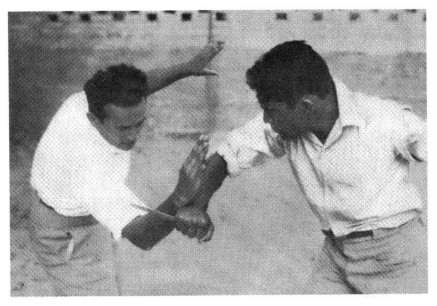

Plate 34.

After he has fallen on his face, move your left hand to help the right hand wrest the dagger from his grasp and kneel on his arm near the shoulder with your left knee. Force him to release his grip on the dagger by pressing strongly on his knuckles. If you have used your left hand to stop the swing, use your right hand to grab his hand from below, twist his hand, and do what is shown in plate 43. In our case, when you grab the hand holding the dagger (not as in the picture), it is much easier because the dagger functions as a lever to twist the attacker's hand.

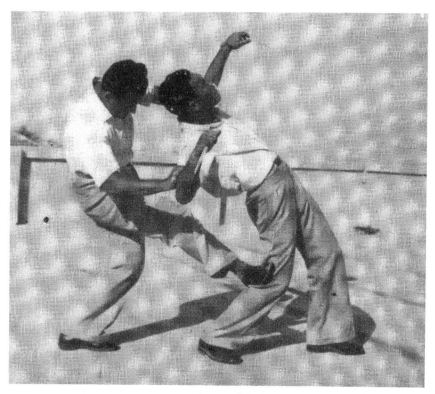

Plate 35.

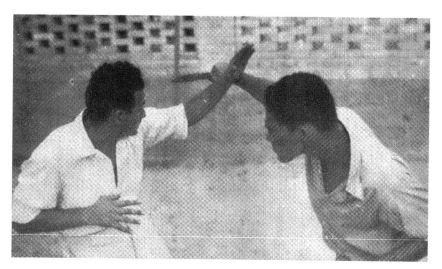

Plate 36.

(85) When attacked, as illustrated in plate 36, and you have stopped his swing with your left hand, wrap your right arm around his arm above the elbow and grab onto your own clothing as high as possible.

Plate 37 illustrates this technique. Try to bring your body behind his arm, as shown in the photo. If you used your right hand to stop his swing, grab the fist holding the dagger so that your thumb is in the direction of the attacker's thumb, then lift it with the help of your left hand. If you have caught the aggressor's fist from below, bring it above your head with a sudden effort and use the momentum to turn easily to your right. This will bring the aggressor to a situation similar to the one shown in plate 52.

Then, keeping your elbows straight, press your right hand into the back of his hand (see plate), causing his fingers to straighten and release the dagger or throw your weight against his hand as shown in plate 53.

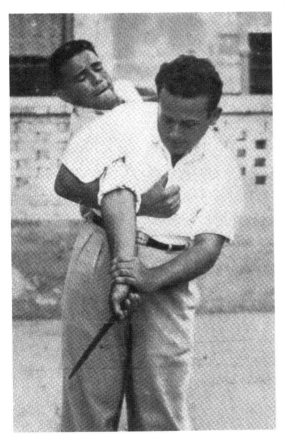

Plate 37.

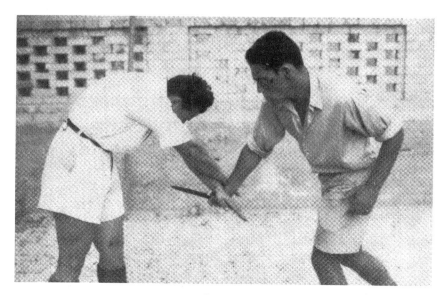

Plate 38.

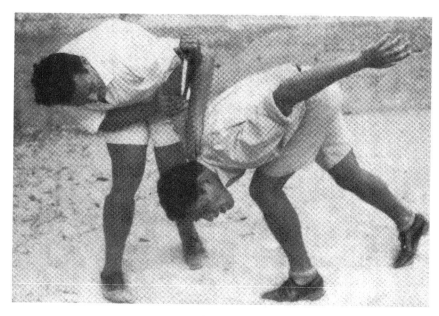

Plate 39.

(86) In the Near East, knife stabs are generally done in an upward motion, "opening the abdomen." The attacker drives his knife in as low as possible and slices the abdomen with a violent effort upwards, as shown in plate 38. Cross your arms, like scissors, so that your right hand is uppermost and trap the attacker's hand between your hands. At first, your arms are slightly bent at the elbow, allowing the hand holding the dagger to get in between but as soon as the dagger hand is between yours, straighten your arms forward and round your back (as shown in the plate) to distance your body from the dagger. Now, using your right hand, grab his sleeve or his arm near the elbow and pull it vigorously towards you while lifting your left hand to his shoulder blade. This produces the situation shown in plate 39. Straighten your left arm, which is holding his clothing or shoulder (as in the plate), and force the attacker to fall on his face. Caution! A dangerous wrench!

(87) If, however, you stopped the attacker's swing with your left hand only, hold his fist so that your thumb is on the back of his fisted hand. Grab his fist from below with your right hand and rotate your hands outwards towards the left. The movement is similar to what the defender is doing to the right in plate 43.

(88) If you stopped the swing with your right hand only, do exactly what is described in section 85. When grabbing the fist that is wielding the dagger, moving slightly forwards and to your right facilitates your defense.

(89) If you have crossed your hands defensively with the left one on top, do not despair. Quickly pull your right hand towards you and continue as if you stopped the swing

with your left hand only. See the previous section [88].

(90) Sometimes using the sounder hand is unavoidable. If the right hand is the sounder hand, take a small step left to shift yourself backward and rapidly interpose your right hand between the knife and the hand

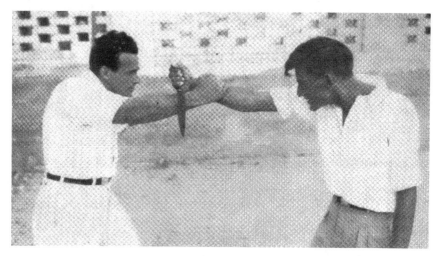

Plate 40.

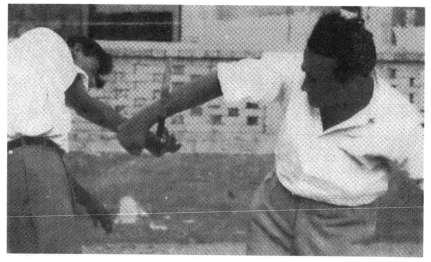

Plate 41.

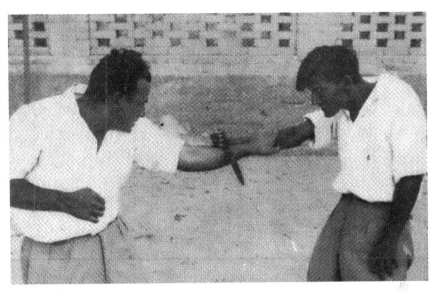

Plate 42.

that is holding it (plate 40). Quickly turn your left shoulder forwards, using your arm as a lever with the hand as the fulcrum. Plate 41 was taken in repose, and actually, the knife will fly up in a large arc and fall to the ground.

(91) If your left hand is the sound one, it is much easier to defend yourself. Stop the thrust as in plate 27 and quickly grab the forearm of the knife-holding hand. As mentioned before, use your arm as a lever while propelling his arm down and lifting your shoulder (see plate 42). The knife will fly out of his hand.

Obviously, it is very easy to cut your hand when using these last two tricks, but this does not lessen their value. With enough level-headedness and deftness, these two stratagems can save you in a truly desperate situation.

(92) When the attacker is merely threatening with a knife, he often brings his empty hand forward. Sometimes

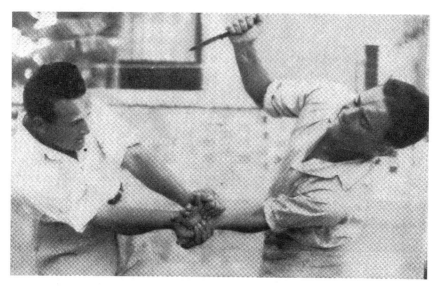

Plate 43.

he will also try grabbing your lapels. There is nothing more effective than holding his thumb (as shown in plate 43) and twisting the entire hand with your other hand. Caution! A movement that is too vehement and severe will dislocate the hand and force him to fall on his nape.

(93) If you initially caught hold of him with your left hand, bring your right hand underneath his armpit and grab his clothing (in plate 44, the hand is not holding onto the shirt because the material is too thin, but this hold is sufficient). Straighten your right arm and press downwards with your left hand. This will cause pain in his elbow and shoulder.

(94) Plate 45 shows how to remove a knife or any other object from a fist. Pressing suddenly, strongly on the fist causes great pain and the hand will not serve its owner for quite a while. Caution!

(95) Plate 46 shows how to defend yourself when lying on the ground. The attacker has already stepped forward with his left leg and grabbed the pants leg on the leg that is poised to kick in an attempt to topple him backward. He will fall and injure his lower spine and neck. After he has fallen, grab his leg, as shown in plate 23. In general, it is possible to use the same tricks while lying on the ground as those used while standing.

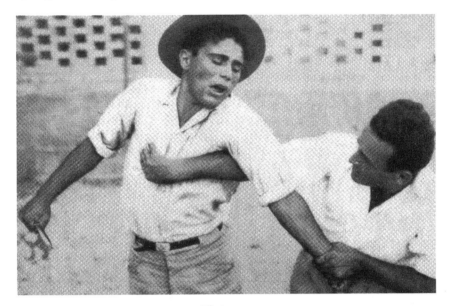

Plate 44.

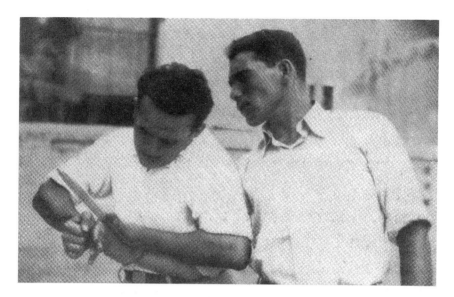

Plate 45.

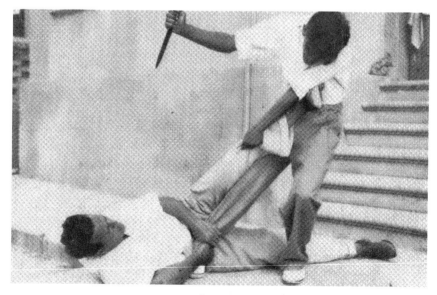

Plate 46.

X. Defending Yourself Against Strangleholds

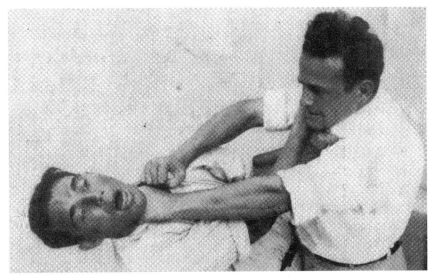

Plate 47.

All strangleholds can be divided into two categories. The first type, where the windpipe is pressed back towards the cervical vertebra, is less painful and takes a relatively long time to cause death (see the stranglehold in plate 54 and the stranglehold with crossed hands in plate 47).

To defend against this type of stranglehold, you must bring the head down towards the chest as far as possible and turn it to one side. The neck muscles contract between the windpipe and the strangler's hands, which lessens the pain.

The second and more dangerous type is where the windpipe is pulled from in front. In this type of stranglehold, the hands are not grasping the whole neck, as in the first instance, but the trachea itself. The important principle here is to steer clear of making an effort with the neck muscles because this will only increase the strangulation. Take a step forward towards the strangler and the strangulation loosens a bit. Attempting to escape by moving backward can rip or tear the vertebra even before the attacker intends this to happen.

A one-handed stranglehold is less dangerous. All the techniques to defend against strangulation are twice as effective against one-handed strangulation so that we will deal only with two-handed strangulation for the sake of brevity.

(96) The strangler is using crossed hands, as in plate 47, holding onto your collar with elbows bent, pressing the backs of his hands or wrists into your throat (a very dangerous strangulation). Grab his collar or shirt to pull him towards you and simultaneously press the knuckles of your other hand, which is holding the other side of his collar, into his throat (see plate 47). Your hand reduces the diameter of the collar and your knuckles displace his throat. Your stranglehold is of the second and more dangerous type and he will immediately loosen his hold on you.

(97) If the strangler is standing behind you and attempting to strangle you using both hands, grab his hands and lift your elbows outwards (see plate 48) to create some free space beneath his pinkies. Insinuate your thumbs under his pinky fingers and hold them firmly; now fold his pinkies backward and turn to your left (for instance, see plate 49). Without loosening your

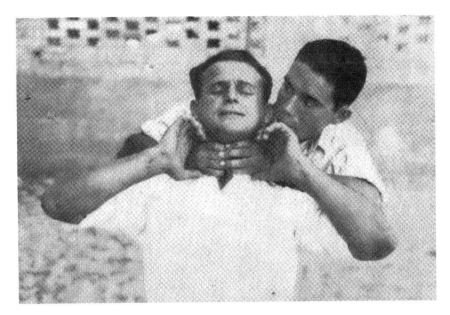

Plate 48.

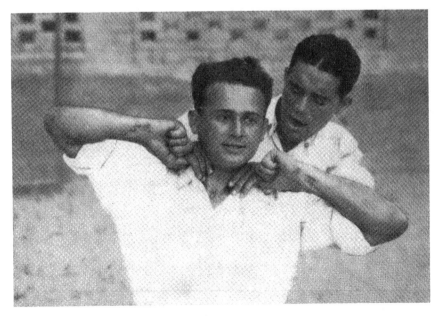

Plate 49.

grip, bring his hands over your head. Your turn crosses his hands, as shown in plate 50. A light pull downwards forces the strangler to fall on his head and shatters his pinky fingers.

(98) If you are being strangled, as shown in plate 51, grab his left hand with your left hand. Then raise your right hand to grab his left hand as well. It is enough to insert the tips of your fingers under the blade of his hand. As shown in the plate, turn your hands and head suddenly to your right, pivoting around his hand; your left elbow lifts and your right elbow lowers. Simultaneously step to the left, behind his left leg. Hold his hand very strongly and don't allow him to remove it from your throat. You will achieve the position shown in plate 52. Pressing on the back of his right hand (as shown in the plate) will bend him to your will. In an effort to relieve the pain, he bends over and you can lean into his hand

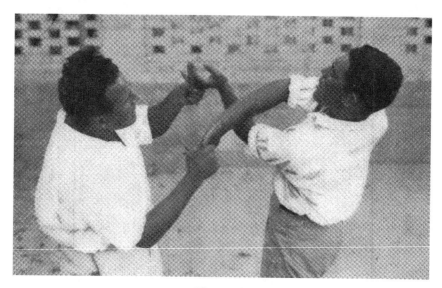

Plate 50.

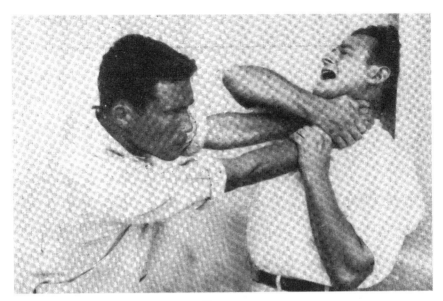

Plate 51.

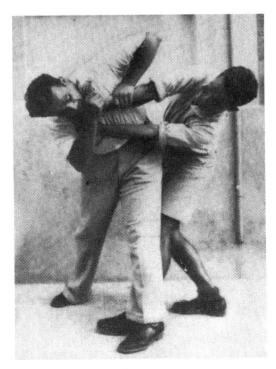

Plate 52.

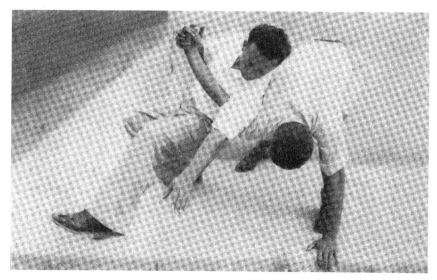

Plate 53.

with your full body weight, as shown in plate 53. Caution!

(99) If you are being strangled, as shown in plate 54, grab his hand, as shown in the picture. Then rapidly push your other hand between his hands in the direction of your head. Do it so that your arms are straight over your head when standing. This will easily distance his left hand from your throat and bring it under your armpit. Grasp his arm at the elbow and grab your forearm with the other hand (see plate 56). Straighten your hands in an easy movement to the right and he will fall off of you so that the arm that you are holding turns you. Your body weight, resisting the turn, will cause him awful pain (see plate 56).

(100) If you are lying on the ground and the strangler is holding you by the throat, rather than by the neck, it is impossible to insinuate your hand between his as this will cause his hand to drag your trachea and you

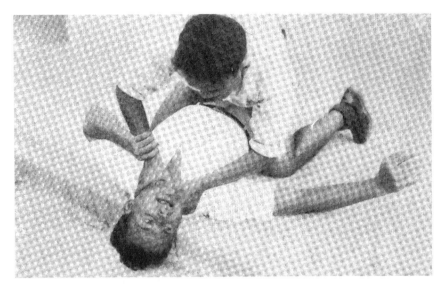

Plate 54.

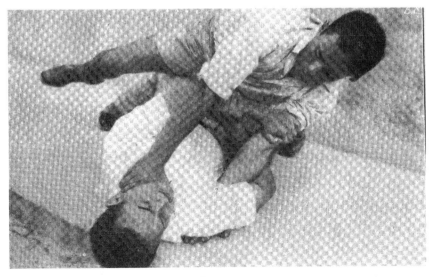

Plate 55.

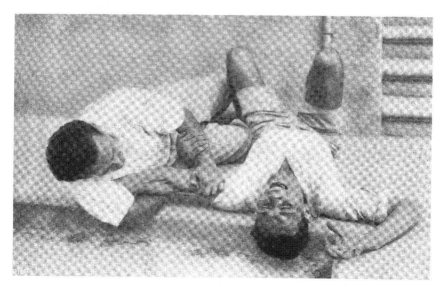

Plate 56.

will choke. In this case, using both hands, grab his left hand as close as possible to the palm (similar to plate 51). Powerfully hoist your left leg over his arm and bring your calf under his chin. Do not relax the pressure on his hand; on the contrary, pull it towards you with all your strength and at the same time straighten your knees. The leg movement chokes him and tilts his body to the side where your leg blocks the tilt. Caution! Strangulation! The trick can also be completed, as shown in plate 66.

XI. Defense Against Firearms and Other Subterfuges and Ploys

It is obvious that hands alone cannot serve as a defense against bullets, but if the gun is used as a threat and the intention is only to rob you, it is entirely possible to thwart his scheme.

To protect yourself, it is better to interrupt when the gun is being drawn rather than when it is already in his hand.

(101) When the attacker moves his hand towards his pocket (it will be the side or back pocket), use your left hand to grab his hand at the wrist and press it towards his body (see plate 57). Insert your other hand into the space between his arm and body and grab his elbow. Vigorously turning his arm backward, pull suddenly to-

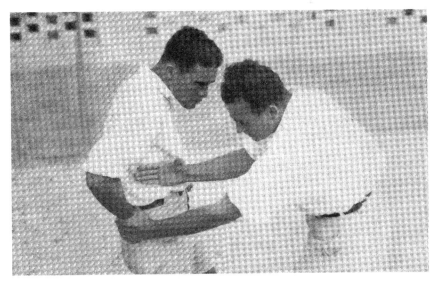

Plate 57.

wards you with your right hand and push his arm up towards his shoulder blade with your left (as shown in plate
58). This can also be completed as shown in plate 39.

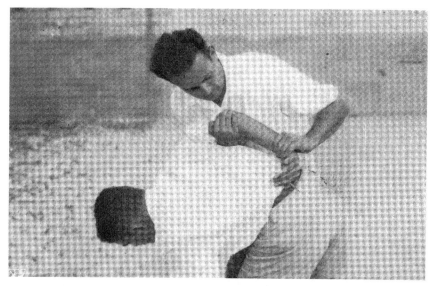

Plate 58.

(102) If the attacker is very strong, it is better to
introduce your right hand into the space between his
hand and body from above and behind his arm. Then
grab his wrist with your left hand as in plate 59. Pushing and twisting the attacker's arm towards his shoulder
blade can force the strongest man to abandon his evil
intentions.

(103) If the aggressor is carrying his gun in a belt
holster, hold the end of the holster containing the bar-
rel of the gun and lift it. If the attacker already has hold
of the gun but hasn't drawn it yet, this will prevent him
from taking it out of the holster; if he hasn't grabbed the
gun yet, this will prevent him from getting hold of it. If

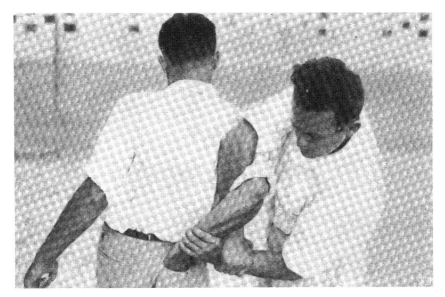

Plate 59.

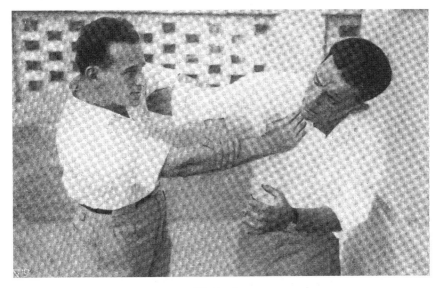

Plate 60.

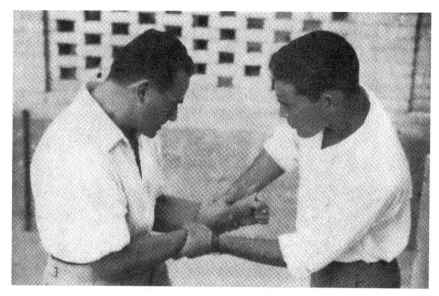

Plate 61.

the holster is hanging on his left, grab with your right hand and use your left hand to strike at him, as shown in plate 25. With your left leg, kick behind his left leg close to the heel (as in plate 62). Your fist's blow and the impetus of your leg will turn him, as shown in plate 21. If your fist lands forcefully exactly on point 3 in plate 24, the attacker loses all sensation. If the attacker has already grabbed the gun, beware not to approach in the direction that a bullet will fly because your movements can cause the gun to fire.

(104) If the attacker has the gun in his hand (at his command, you raised your hands), stare directly into his eyes as he is advancing towards you. Then like a bolt out of the blue, use your left hand to strike the hand holding the gun diagonally and down—away from you. With your other hand, strike point 2 in plate 24 with all your might. This is similar to plate 26. You can also complete the

maneuver, as shown in plate 60. Wrap your hand (after moving the gun aside by striking it as described) around his hand and use your other hand to grab and press his hand towards his chest, preventing him from transferring the gun to his other hand. You can also complete this maneuver, as shown in plate 37 and the first part of section 85.

(105) Plates 61 and 62 show how to free both arms at the same time. Turn your hands until you see the assailant's fingernails. Bring your elbows together in front of

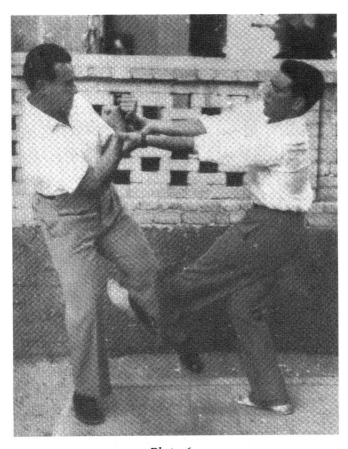

Plate 62.

your chest and then bring your body towards your hands so that your elbows bend more, thus providing more power. Lean backward a bit while you straighten your body, letting one fist help the other (see plate 62). Kick his weight-bearing leg, to which he shifted his weight when you brought your elbows together, from behind. He will fall, and, in any case, he will release your arms.

(106) If he is holding one of your arms with both hands, as shown in plate 63, make a fist and grab it with your other hand. With a strong impetus (use your whole body), lift your hands and bring them to the other side of your body. At the same time, kick the back of his left leg with your right foot. The momentum of your arms is in the opposite direction of the leg's momentum and he will fall to the ground like a sheaf of grain.

(107) If the attacker is very strong and the area has a soft surface (such as sand or plowed earth), it is best to do thusly: with your free hand, grab one of his hands and strongly pull your hands towards you. At the same time, butt him in the face, the nose, or the lower teeth.

(108) If he is holding your arm with both hands, introduce your free hand between his hands and grab your trapped hand that you have balled into a fist. Pull your fist towards you while leaning all your weight onto the trapped arm, which is bent at the elbow in a straight angle. Your hand will be freed easily, even if his grip is much stronger than yours. Also, try to trip him as in previous exercises or immediately strike a sharp, quick blow at point 3 in plate 24.

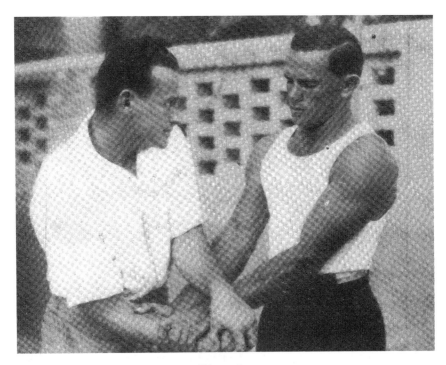

Plate 63.

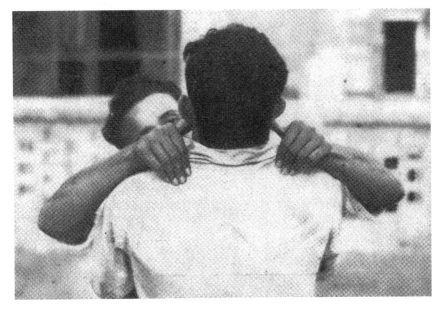

Plate 64.

(109) Plate 64 shows how to apply pressure on point 2 in plate 24, which frees you from all sorts of frontal clinches and holds that leave your arms are free. If your arms are trapped between his body and yours, butt him in the face with your forehead and at the same time stomp his toe (point 11 in plate 24) with the heel of your shoe. You can also transfer one of your hands, so they are both on the same side. Lean all your weight onto your assailant via the shoulder of the hand that crossed over. Then with the leg on the leaning side (on the side where both your hands are), kick the attacker's leg from behind. He will release you as he falls. If he does not release you, he will sustain an even greater injury when your entire body weight lands on him.

(110) Plates 65 and 66 show how to defend yourself and subdue the assailant who has thrown you to the ground and is punching your face. Grab hold of his clothing with one hand, so he can't get away from you. Position the fingers of your other hand under his nose and push towards his back using a sawing motion. (Notice the position of the fingers covering his mouth; if your fingers are parallel to his mouth, they are in danger of being bitten). Push his head between your spread, raised legs and cross your ankles, making a great effort to squeeze them together (see plate 66). Grab his arm as it moves backward and bring it sideways towards your hip with his palm is facing upwards. Now press on it. Caution! You can break his arm!

(111) In addition to the squeeze described in item 109 and plate 64, there are many grips that are very painful if your fingers are trained to grip strongly. Holding

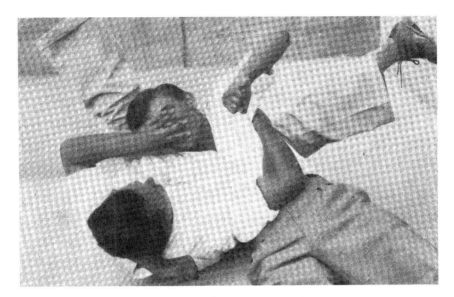

Plate 65.

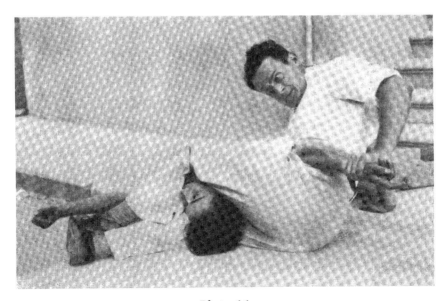

Plate 66.

his shoulder, at the point marked 5 in plate 24, dig your thumb into the muscle and squeeze strongly with your fingers. He will writhe and thrash about from the pain. If you grip these muscles strongly on either side of the neck, it is possible to force him to the ground. The pain is intense and does not immediately let up when you loosen your grip.

(112) Extremely painful spots are found a few centimeters below the point marked 2 in plate 24. Putting a finger here, just under the lower jaw, and pushing forward and up in the direction of the ear will immediately free you from his bear hug.

(113) If your arms free because he has caught you from behind, spread your legs, bend forward, and grab one of his ankles. Then pull upwards, leaning your weight on the thigh of the leg you are holding. He will fall backward and release you. After he falls, grab the heel of his shoe with your right hand (assuming you initially grabbed his right ankle) or, if he is barefoot, grab the leg itself, and twist his leg so that the toes point inwards (the opposite direction of how Charlie Chaplin turns his feet). If you initially grabbed his left ankle, then use your left hand to grab his left heel, etc. It is helpful to stand on his other calf, close to the ankle, giving him no choice but to surrender.

(114) If he has lifted you off the ground, hold both of his arms so that he cannot suddenly separate them. Then vigorously straighten your body, smashing your head into his face. Or lean your hands on his arms, so you push them into the curve between his thighs and hips. Lift both your legs forward and spread and bring them

down forcefully, grabbing his ankles. Then continue as in stratagem 113.

(115) If he has grabbed you from behind and lifted you in a way that neutralizes your arms, then place one foot behind the knee of your other leg and move your other foot in between the attacker's legs, put it behind his leg (which is on the side of your bent leg) at ankle height. Make an effort with that leg and, at the same time, move the bent knee back and out. He will fall backward. The leg action is similar to that of the hands in plate 56. You can also free yourself from this situation by crossing your left foot behind your right heel between the legs of your assailant. Bend your right leg and lift it so that the heel of your shoe is between his knee and your left leg and against his knee joint. Then stomp vigorously. His leg will twist outwards and bend at the knee, forcing him to let go of you or fall to the ground. If the stomp is sudden and strong enough, his knee locks and the tendons of the lateral muscles stretch.

(116) It is better to bend your knees and dig your heels into the ground. The attacker will surely take advantage of the opportunity and throw you to the ground. This maneuver lifts his arms and brings them closer to your shoulders. Abruptly stretch your arms forward and his hands will slide off of you completely. At this moment, his body is tilted forward, so clasp his knees and pull him towards you. Your shoulders stop the forward motion of his legs and your hands become a strong lever, causing him to fall on his face. Spread your legs when you pull, so he falls onto the ground and not onto your legs. Continue the movement of your hands and shoul-

ders until his shins begin to fold towards his thighs. Your interlocked hands are now behind his knees, preventing his shins from coming close to his thighs. Your shoulders, which are now pressing on his feet, cause him severe pain in the ankles and knees. It is like the trick described in plate 23, but much more powerful.

(117) If your attacker is holding your clothing or collar in front, grab his clothing as close to his head as possible. Pick one leg up, bent at all its joints, and brace it against his pubic bone or a little higher on his lower abdomen. Pull him forcefully towards you and, at the same time, fold your other leg under yourself. You will fall to the ground, falling backward as described in plate 17, although your hands are not on the ground. You will not be injured by the fall because your assailant curbs your fall, so you fall easily to the ground. The foot that is resting against the attacker's body should be turned with the toes outward, so his center of gravity is against the middle of your foot and he cannot slide off your foot. Raise his hips and his entire lower body and roll over your head by straightening the leg and making an effort with your hands. If you let go of him immediately after pushing your leg up, he will fall on his head. Caution! This fall can be fatal.

(118) There are those who attack from behind, grabbing the head so that the bend of the elbow is right under the chin and the other hand is holding the fist of the arm that is strangling you. If the attacker is smart enough to turn so that his hip is against your backside, it is enough for him to bend forward a little and you will be hanging with your throat over his arm, chok-

ing. First, using the arm that is between you and him, grab the sleeve near the shoulder of the strangling hand. This movement alleviates the weight and allows you to get some air. Now grab his pants at the inseam, near his knee, suddenly turn your entire body, so your leg (on the side holding his pants) comes behind his leg. While turning, pull both hands together (the one holding the sleeve to your chest and the other hand) and upwards; thus, one hand helps the other. Even if the person strangling you is very heavy, you will still succeed in subduing him and forcing him to the ground. If he is not very heavy, you can shake him and roll him over your back by vigorously tugging his sleeve and turning your body to lean his body against yours.

Closing Comments

The Japanese teach many more strategies. However, a man needs to study and acquire the requisite patience and steadiness that the Japanese have in order to make them useful. Even then, if a person neglects his training for a fairly long time, his maneuvers will not be serviceable. We have presented some of the moves in an unusual form, one that is suitable for self defense. In their usual form, these maneuvers are more like a circus act or entertainment played for the pleasure of the audience.

ABOUT MOSHE FELDENKRAIS, D.SC.[38, 39]

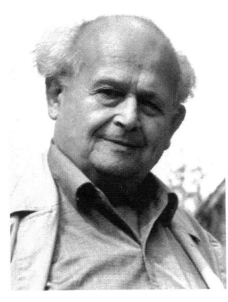

Moshe Feldenkrais, D.Sc. (1904-1984). Photo courtesy of *Feldenkrais* Institute Tel Aviv, Israel.

The *Feldenkrais Method* was developed by Dr. Moshe Feldenkrais (1904 – 1984).

Moshe Feldenkrais (Doctor of Science, Sorbonne) was an engineer, physicist, inventor, martial artist, and student of human development. Born in Slavuta, present-day Ukraine, to a distinguished family known as high-quality publishers of Jewish publications, he emigrated as a Zionist at age fourteen to Palestine, where he worked as a laborer, studied martial arts, and completed his high school at age twenty-three—with honors. After working as a cartographer for the British survey office, he left for France. He graduated in 1933 from the Ècole de Traveaux Publics de Paris in Mechanical and Electrical Engineering. Later, he studied at the Sorbonne while working under Frederic Joliot-Curie at the Radium Institute in Paris. His interest in Jiu-Jitsu brought him into contact with Professor Jigoro Kano, who developed Judo. Dr. Feldenkrais was a founder of the Jiu-Jitsu Club of Paris and was one of the first Europeans to earn a black belt in Judo (1936).

Escaping the Nazi advance, he went to Britain and worked on anti-submarine research for the British Admiralty. It was there, in the forties, motivated by his attempts to heal a recurring knee injury first sustained while playing soccer in 1929 and uncertain prospects for surgery, that he began to develop his Method and wrote his first book on the subject. Thus began for Feldenkrais a life-long exploration of the relationship between movement and consciousness. In the fifties, Dr. Feldenkrais returned to Israel, where he lived and taught his Method that has now spread worldwide. He died in 1984 in Tel Aviv, Israel.

In developing his work, Moshe Feldenkrais studied, among other things, anatomy, physiology, child development, movement science, evolution, psychology, and several Eastern awareness practices and other somatic approaches.

Dr. Feldenkrais authored several seminal books on movement, learning, human consciousness, and somatic experience. He taught in Israel and Europe through the sixties and seventies and North America through the seventies and eighties. He trained his first group of teachers in Tel Aviv in the early seventies. He then led two groups in the USA—one group in San Francisco, California, and another in Amherst, Massachusetts.

Dr. Feldenkrais worked with and helped tens of thousands of people with functional movement disorders in his life. His work's focus was using movement and the accompanying sensation of movement as the vehicle by which his students learned and perfected their functional abilities; hence he called his work *Awareness through Movement*. By providing an enormous range of learning experiences to people of all ages and disabilities, he freed them from restrictions imposed by static medical diagnoses. He helped heads of state such as David ben Gurion and Moshe Dayan, artists such as Yehudi Menhuhin, sports figures such as Dr. J., children with cerebral palsy, and countless others.

He taught over some years for the dramatist Peter Brook and his Théâtre Bouffes du Nord. He was a collaborator with anthropologist Margaret Mead, neuroscientist Karl Pribram, and explorers of the psychophysical Jean Houston and Robert Masters.

The breadth, vitality, and precision of Dr. Feldenkrais's work has seen it applied in fields as diverse as neurology, psychology, performing arts, sports, and rehabilitation.

ABOUT MOTI (MORDEHAI) NATIV

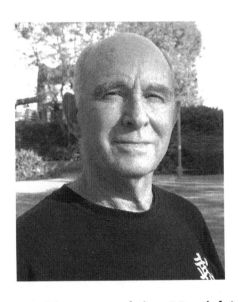

Moti (Mordehai) Nativ, a retired colonel from the Israel Defense Forces, is a certified teacher of the *Feldenkrais Method* and Martial Arts.

Moti has graduated from the Jerusalem 1 *Feldenkrais* Professional Practitioner training in 1994 and served as the president of the Israeli *Feldenkrais* Guild.

Moti began studying Martial Arts in 1966, and his martial arts practice includes wrestling, Judo and Krav Maga. He holds a black belt in Judo, and he is a certified Krav Maga instructor.

Moti is Dai Shihan (master teacher) of Bujinkan school of Budo TaiJutsu. He is a member of this school since 1975, and since 1995 he has led the training of Bujinkan teachers in Israel. He founded the Bujinkan Shiki (Awareness) Dojo.

About Moti (Mordehai) Nativ

Moti has explored the peculiar way that brought Moshe Feldenkrais from the Land of Israel to become a Judo Master in France and England and the influence of the Martial Arts on the development of the *Feldenkrais Method*.

Moti teaches advanced workshops called, *"The Synergy of Martial Arts and the Feldenkrais Method"* worldwide.

Moti republished Moshe Feldenkrais's book *Practical Unarmed Combat* (originally published in 1942) and was involved in republishing *Higher Judo* (1948) and *Autosuggestion* (1929). Lately, he published an article about Moshe's unique work *Better Judo* (1948-1949).

ENDNOTES

1. Eretz Yisrael – The Land of Israel. The 1917 Balfour Declaration announced British support for the establishment of a Jewish homeland. It inspired many Jews to uproot themselves from their homes, fleeing from the rising anti-Semitism and murderous pogroms in Europe, and make their way to Eretz Yisrael. Moshe Feldenkrais arrived in Eretz Yisrael in 1919 at a pivotal point in world history. The Ottoman Empire had conceded the area of Eretz Yisrael to the British at the end of WWI in 1918. A League of Nations mandate, which went into effect in July 1920, ended the British military administration of the territory and granted the British civil administration of the area they called Palestine-Eretz Yisrael. Turbulent times indeed. I have often wondered about his journey. And how young Moshe Feldenkrais, who set out from his home to travel to an unknown land, envisioned his destination. What image did he have in his mind? Did his destination have a name? He was well versed in the history of his people and was conversant with texts that expressed the longing of an exiled people for its homeland; Psalm 137 (written circa 539 BCE), "By the rivers of Babylon, there we sat down, yea, we wept, when we remembered Zion." Zion – a synonym for the Land of Israel – Eretz Yisrael.

2. I wrote the foreword for *Thinking and Doing* (2013), the English edition of Feldenkrais' translation of *Autosuggestion*, where I spoke about Feldenkrais' basic concept for his self-defense method.

3. A literal translation of the Hebrew is "face-to-face combat".

4. In 1976, Eli Avikzar was appointed as the head of Krav Maga in the IDF. I was trained by him to become a military Krav Maga instructor.

5. Amherst, 1981.

6. Hillel, Pirkei Avot (Ethics of the Ancestors) 1:14.

7. The Hebrew word "aliya" means ascent or rise, but for generations it has been used to mean "to immigrate to the

Land of Israel". The third Aliya (1919 – 1923) consisted mainly of young people from eastern Europe and spurred by the Russian October Revolution and the ensuing anti-Semitic pogroms.

8. Quote from an interview in San Francisco, 1977.

9. This quote appears in the draft version I discovered in the Kodokan archives. Even though the volume you are holding pre-dates the Kodokan version, I have taken the liberty of quoting from the later version.

10. *Criminal Investigation by Prof Hans Gross* (Translator's Note (TN) – This was a footnote in the original text).

11. A teacher or instructor in Japanese martial arts; a master.

12. Amherst interview.

13. KAPAP, a Hebrew acronym for Krav Panim el Panim, is a close-quarter battle system of defensive tactics, hand-to-hand combat, and self-defense. (Wikipedia)

14. The Defense of the Weak Against the Aggressor.

15. In that era "oriental" indicated the Near East. In today's parlance it means the Middle East.

16. Moshe Feldenkrais, *Judo: The Art of Defense and Attack*, England, 1941.

17. The Kodokan Judo Institute, founded by Jigoro Kano and located in Tokyo, is the headquarters of the international Judo community and houses a large collection of archival material.

18. Catch wrestling (also known as Catch-As-Catch-Can and Strong Style) is a hybrid grappling style and combat sport. It was developed by J. G. Chambers in Britain circa 1870 and popularized by wrestlers of traveling fun fairs. Catch wrestling derives from various different international styles of wrestling. The training of some modern professional wrestlers and mixed martial artists is founded in catch wrestling. (Wikipedia)

19. William James (1842-1910), American philosopher and psychologist.

20. In *Higher Judo* he uses the term the "Art of Falling".

21. One of Emil's famous fights was when he bested Muhamad Nagib, the Egyptian army champion, who later became to be the president of the Egypt.

22. https://www.youtube.com/watch?v=z_ITiwOeFdw&ab_channel=ThomGoddard

23. San Francisco – 1975 Week 1, Day 1, 16 June, afternoon.

24. Rabbi Hillel (c. 30 BCE – 9 CE). The quotation is from Pirkei Avot ii.4.

25. An exhortation that appears many times in the Torah.

26. This phrase appears numerous times in the Torah in myriad contexts.

27. *Criminal Investigation* by Prof Hans Gross (TN – This was a footnote in the original text.)

28. See *A General Introduction to Psychoanalysis* by Sigmund Freud. (TN – This was a footnote in the original text.)

29. How to wean yourself from fear, consult *The Practice of Autosuggestion: By the Method of Emile Coue* by S.H. Brooks, translated and annotated by the author of this book. (TN – This was a footnote in the original text.)

30. The German and English phrases appear in the original. (TN)

31. This statement might not be as specious as it sounds. It is only recently that education system stopped forcing left-handed children into right handedness. It therefore follows that in a society where school was not compulsory, left-handed people remained left handed.

32. Modern Hebrew was in the process of evolving, so these terms were probably not yet definitively determined. Translator's note.

33. In the Bible, God commands the Priests (Kohanim) to bless the Children of Israel. The verses of the Priestly Blessing (Birkat Kohanim) are among the oldest in continuous

liturgical use. Archaeologists found the words etched on silver scrolls found in tombs from the seventh century BCE. The words of the Priestly Blessing come from the Book of Numbers 6:24-26. "May the Lord bless you and keep you. May the Lord let His face shine upon you and be gracious unto you. May the Lord look kindly upon you and give you peace." The hands are held together palms-down with the fingers split so there are 5 spaces: one space between the thumbs, a space between the thumb and first finger of each hand, and a space between the second and third finger of each hand. This hand gesture has been popularized by the Star Trek television series, as the Vulcan ritual of greeting. (TN)

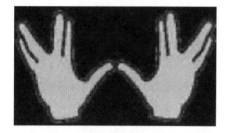

34. "Monday and Thursday" is a colloquial expression meaning "routinely". It originates in the Yiddish expression, which has its roots in the tradition of reading a short section of the week's Torah portion on Mondays and Thursdays, in addition to the full reading on Saturdays. (TN)

35. This sentence appears in English in the original. (TN)

36. Appears in German in the original. (TN)

37. Appears in English in the original. (TN)

38. Mark Reese, 1951 – 2006. Author of *Moshe Feldenkrais - A Life in Movement, Volume 1*.

39. IFF Materials Website. Moshe Feldenkrais Biography, http://feldenkrais-method.org/en/biography.

RESOURCES

For information about *Feldenkrais* products, classes, courses, articles and other resources:
The *Feldenkrais* Store
AchievingExcellence.com

For information about *Feldenkrais* in Practice, Moti Nativ's Method visit: Feldenkrais-IP.org

For information about *Feldenkrais Method*, *Feldenkrais* practitioners and professional trainings, contact the *Feldenkrais Guild* of North America:
FeldenkraisGuild.com

To find *Feldenkrais* practitioners and classes in your area visit: Feldenkrais.com

The Israeli *Feldenkrais* Guild: Feldenkrais-Israel.org

International *Feldenkrais* Federation:
Feldenkrais-Method.org